the blender bible

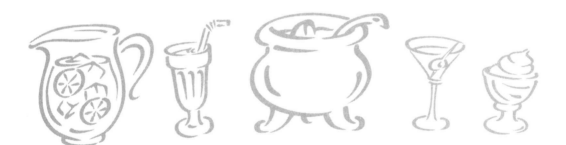

Andrew Chase & Nicole Young

Robert
ROSE

The Blender Bible
Text copyright © 2005 Andrew Chase and Nicole Young
Photographs copyright © 2005 Robert Rose Inc.
Cover and text design copyright © 2005 Robert Rose Inc.

For complete cataloguing information, see page 367.

Disclaimer
The recipes in this book have been carefully tested by our kitchen and our tasters. To the best of our knowledge, they are safe and nutritious for ordinary use and users. For those people with food or other allergies, or who have special food requirements or health issues, please read the suggested contents of each recipe carefully and determine whether or not they may create a problem for you. All recipes are used at the risk of the consumer.

We cannot be responsible for any hazards, loss or damage that may occur as a result of any recipe use.

For those with special needs, allergies, requirements or health problems, in the event of any doubt, please contact your medical adviser prior to the use of any recipe.

Design & Production: PageWave Graphics Inc.
Editor: Sue Sumeraj
Recipe Tester: Jennifer MacKenzie
Proofreader: Sheila Wawanash
Index: Gillian Watts
Photography: Mark T. Shapiro
Food Styling: Kate Bush
Props Styling: Charlene Erricson
Color Scans & Film: Rayment & Collins

Front cover image: Quick Hummus (see recipe, page 24), Fresh Pea and Arugula Soup (see recipe, page 110), Frozen Berry Daiquiri (see recipe, page 244) and Mango Ginger Smoothie (see recipe, page 215).

We acknowledge the financial support of the Government of Canada through the Book Publishing Industry Development Program (BPIDP) for our publishing activities.

Published by Robert Rose Inc.
120 Eglinton Avenue East, Suite 800, Toronto, Ontario, Canada M4P 1E2
Tel: (416) 322-6552 Fax: (416) 322-6936

Printed in Canada

1 2 3 4 5 6 7 8 9 CPL 12 11 10 09 08 07 06 05

Contents

Acknowledgments

This book is a collaborative project. The imaginative scope of the recipes would have been impossible to produce without the help of two of my colleagues. Gabrielle Bright, formerly my sous-chef and restaurant partner and now recipe developer at the Canadian Living Test Kitchen, and Annabelle Waugh, of the Canadian Living Test Kitchen and an indispensable and highly valued member of the Homemakers Test Kitchen, contributed recipes and helped in the discussions of the scope of the book. I am beholden to them for their assistance.

Thanks also to Cuisinart for supplying the blenders we used in testing these recipes. The SmartPower™ 7-Speed Electronic is a first-class blender — durable, versatile and easy to clean. It will give you great performance for years.

I thank publisher Bob Dees for suggesting the project to me. Sue Sumeraj has been an excellent editor. I must also thank my partner, Camilo Costales, for steering clear of me and remaining patient during the sometimes hectic writing of this book. Great thanks to my friends and neighbors for selflessly helping me taste the results of the recipe development and seldom complaining about all the smooth food.

— Andrew Chase

I have to thank Liam and Claire for being my inspiration to make baby food and David for giving me our inspirations and providing the time, support and encouragement to finish this book. I love you all more than food! It was the ideal year for taste testers, as we had eleven babies born to friends, and I am very appreciative of all the discerning palates. May you all be healthy eaters with massive appetites!

Thanks to Andrew for recommending me, publisher Bob Dees for giving me the project, and my lawyer, sister and friend Danielle for looking out for me since we were little. Thanks also to my sister Stephanie for her blender wisdom. I'd like to express my gratitude to Nadine Day, registered dietitian extraordinaire, for her advice and nutritional analysis, and to Judy Coveney for introducing us. Thanks to Sue Sumeraj, our patient editor, for teaching me the process and making me seem literate.

Finally, eternal thanks to my mom and dad for showing me what it means to be a great parent and teaching me that anything is possible.

— Nicole Young

Introduction

With the introduction of the household blender in the 1930s, blenders became a fixture in North American kitchens. But since the popularization of food processors in the '70s, blenders have been gradually and mistakenly relegated to the status of mere beverage mixers, and their many other uses have been neglected. Blenders are an indispensable and extremely convenient kitchen tool. From grinding spices to puréeing soups to mixing beverages to making batter, blenders help keep your cooking on a smooth track. So find your blender a place on the kitchen counter!

In my many years as restaurant chef and recipe writer, I have learned to depend on the blender. Nothing grinds large batches of spices like a blender, and no other tool can chop harder ingredients, such as lemon grass, to a fine, digestible consistency. Blenders allow you to make wonderful homemade peanut butter, mayonnaise and pepper purée. Dips, spreads and simple pasta sauces such as tomato sauce and pesto become a breeze; soups can be puréed in seconds. Curry pastes no longer require strenuous and time-consuming work with a mortar and pestle — many Indian households in North America now rely heavily on the blender for food preparation. Healthy breakfast drinks and quick desserts are a bonus.

Blenders are extremely useful in basic food preparation:

- Making bread crumbs: Break stale and dry bread into small pieces by hand. Pulse in 1-cup (250 mL) batches to desired consistency. (You can make cookie and cracker crumbs the same way.)
- Grating hard cheese: Cube cheese in $1/2$-inch (1 cm) pieces. Blend on high speed in $1/2$-cup (125 mL) batches.
- Grinding coffee: Grind coffee on high speed in 1-cup (250 mL) batches until desired consistency.
- Grinding spices: Grind spices on high speed in $1/4$-cup (50 mL) to $1/2$-cup (125 mL) batches until desired consistency.
- Whipping cream: Whip 1 cup (250 mL) cream on low speed until thick and smooth.
- Chopping nuts: Pulse $1/2$ cup (125 mL) to 1 cup (250 mL) nuts several times, scraping down sides with a spatula between each pulsing.
- Making mushroom powder: Break up 1 oz (30 g) dried mushrooms into small pieces by hand. Pulse on high speed to a fine powder. Use as a seasoning in sauces to give a rich mushroom flavor.
- Preparing dried tomato paste: Pour $3/4$ cup (175 mL) boiling water over 1 oz (30 g) dried (oven-dried or sun-dried) tomatoes. Let stand until soft, about 20 minutes. Purée on high speed until smooth, then strain through fine sieve. Use this sweet and intensely flavored purée in place of tomato paste.

When using your blender, you may be concerned about which speed to use. In this book, I have chosen to simplify the speed question by indicating only low or high speeds. In general, low speed is ideal for finely chopping ingredients. High speed makes fine purées. When high-speed blending is indicated, you might want to start on a lower speed and increase to high when ingredients are finely chopped. To avoid spillage when blending at high speed, fill the blender only half-full (this is especially important with hot ingredients). If your blender has intermediate speeds, you can experiment to see which speed works best for the food at hand. There is no magic about it: longer blending at a lower speed will give pretty much the same results as shorter blending at high speed. Whenever you use your blender, stop it partway through blending to see if the ingredients need to be scraped down with a spatula. This will ensure that the ingredients are evenly blended.

To clean your blender, fill it with hot water and let it run for about 1 minute. Then put it in the dishwasher or wash by hand. Or, if your blender base unscrews from the jug, disassemble it, wash the components separately and allow them to dry thoroughly before reassembling.

In this book, you will find an eclectic collection of excellent recipes, inspired by food from around the world. I have chosen to exclude recipes in which the blender could have been used but isn't an indispensable tool — each recipe in the book requires a blender to produce the best results.

You will undoubtedly discover even more uses for your blender as you cook with these recipes. I hope you find inspiration and surprises in these pages!

— Andrew Chase

Appetizers, Dips and Spreads

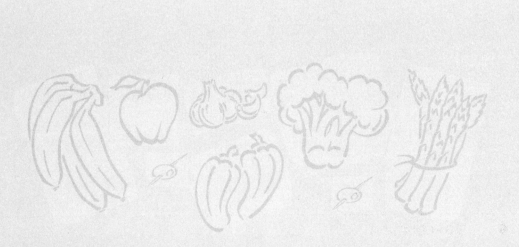

*This popular treat is
easy to make with the
help of the blender.*

Welsh Rarebit

1 cup	ale or stout	250 mL
1 ½ cups	cubed extra-old Cheddar cheese (8 oz/250 g)	375 mL
1	egg yolk	1
½ cup	roughly chopped sweet onions	125 mL
2 tbsp	hot English or Dijon mustard	25 mL
1 tsp	Worcestershire sauce	5 mL
½ tsp	sweet paprika	2 mL
¼ tsp	hot pepper sauce	1 mL
10	slices bread, toasted	10
¼ cup	chopped chives	50 mL

1. In a medium saucepan, bring ale to boil.

2. Meanwhile, in blender, blend cheese, yolk and onions until fine. With motor running, through hole in top, pour in ale, mustard, Worcestershire sauce, paprika and hot pepper sauce. Blend on low speed until smooth. Return to saucepan over medium-high heat. Cook, stirring, for 2 to 3 minutes, until mixture is as thick as heavy cream and coats the back of a spoon.

3. Cut toast in half to make triangles. Arrange on a platter and cover with hot rarebit mixture. Sprinkle with chives.

These cheese croûtes from the francophone part of Switzerland are an undeniably rich treat and typical of that country's cheese cuisine.

TIP

For an even richer flavor, substitute Vacherin cheese from Fribourg or Appenzeller cheese for the Gruyère.

Cheese Croûtes

- Preheat oven to 500°F (260°C)
- Rimmed baking sheet

6	slices crusty white bread or 12 slices baguette	6
⅔ cup	dry white wine, divided	150 mL
3 cups	cubed Gruyère cheese (about 10 oz/300 g)	750 mL
1	whole egg	1
1	egg yolk	1
1	clove garlic, smashed	1
2 tbsp	all-purpose flour	25 mL
Pinch	cayenne pepper	Pinch
¼ tsp	freshly ground black pepper (or to taste)	1 mL

1. On baking sheet, lightly toast bread in preheated oven for about 6 minutes, turning halfway through. Remove from oven and sprinkle with 3 tbsp (45 mL) of the wine. Set aside.

2. In blender, on low speed, blend cheese until shredded. Add remaining wine, egg, egg yolk, garlic, flour and cayenne; blend until fairly smooth.

3. Top toast with cheese mixture and sprinkle with freshly ground pepper. Return to oven and bake until golden, about 10 minutes.

*These simple,
traditional Russian
pancakes are
wonderful topped with
caviar, smoked salmon
or other smoked fish,
gravlax, sour cream
and many other hors
d'oeuvres toppings.*

TIP

Make sure you use
regular buckwheat
flour (sometimes sold
as light buckwheat
flour), not the dark
variety.

Buckwheat Blinis

1 ½ tsp	granulated sugar, divided	7 mL
¼ cup	warm water	50 mL
1 ½ tsp	active dry yeast	7 mL
1	egg	1
1 ½ cups	lukewarm milk	375 mL
¼ cup	butter, melted, divided	50 mL
1 cup	all-purpose flour	250 mL
¾ cup	buckwheat flour	175 mL
½ tsp	salt	2 mL

1. In blender, dissolve ½ tsp (2 mL) of the sugar in warm water. Sprinkle in yeast and let stand until frothy, about 10 minutes. Add egg, milk, 2 tbsp (25 mL) of the butter and the remaining 1 tsp (5 mL) sugar; blend on low speed until frothy. With motor running, through hole in top, gradually add all-purpose flour, buckwheat flour and salt; blend, scraping down sides as necessary, until thoroughly mixed. Scrape into a bowl, cover and let rise in a warm place until doubled in bulk, about 1 hour.

2. Heat a nonstick skillet over medium heat and brush lightly with some of the remaining butter. Without stirring, spoon in batter by scant 2 tablespoonfuls (25 mL), adding butter as necessary. Cook until bubbles form on top that do not fill in, about 1 minute. Turn and cook until bottom is golden, about 30 seconds. Remove to a warmed platter and repeat with remaining batter.

White Flour Blinis

*These blinis are fluffier
than buckwheat blinis
and can be used in the
same manner.*

1 ½ tsp	granulated sugar, divided	7 mL
¼ cup	warm water	50 mL
1 ½ tsp	active dry yeast	7 mL
2	eggs, separated	2
1 ½ cups	lukewarm milk	375 mL
¼ cup	butter, melted, divided	50 mL
2 cups	all-purpose flour	500 mL
½ tsp	salt	2 mL

1. In blender, dissolve ½ tsp (2 mL) of the sugar in warm water. Sprinkle in yeast and let stand until frothy, about 10 minutes. Add egg yolks, milk, 2 tbsp (25 mL) of the butter and the remaining 1 tsp (5 mL) sugar; blend on low speed until frothy. With motor running, through hole in top, gradually add flour and salt; blend, scraping down sides as necessary, until thoroughly mixed. Scrape into a bowl, cover and let rise in a warm place until doubled in bulk, about 1 hour.

2. In clean blender, on high speed, beat egg whites until stiff. Gently fold into batter. Cover and let rest for 15 minutes.

3. Heat a nonstick skillet over medium heat and brush lightly with some of the remaining butter. Without stirring, spoon in batter by scant 2 tablespoonfuls (25 mL), adding butter as necessary. Cook until bubbles form on top that do not fill in, about 1 minute. Turn and cook until bottom is golden, about 30 seconds. Remove to a warmed platter and repeat with remaining batter.

TIPS

It is easier to remove the rind of the Oka cheese if it is cold.

For the best flavor, use unpasteurized Oka Classique. If Oka cheese is unavailable, replace it with Port Salut from France.

Oka Cheese Pots

● *6 ramekins*

1 cup	cubed rindless Oka Classique cheese	250 mL
1 cup	dry cottage cheese (farmer's cheese)	250 mL
½ cup	sour cream	125 mL
⅓ cup	crumbled blue cheese	75 mL
⅓ cup	dry sherry	75 mL
2 tbsp	grated sweet onion	25 mL
2 tbsp	chopped fresh parsley	25 mL
¼ tsp	freshly ground black pepper	1 mL
Pinch	ground cloves	Pinch
Pinch	ground nutmeg	Pinch

1. In blender, on low speed, blend Oka cheese, cottage cheese, sour cream, blue cheese, sherry, onion, parsley, pepper, cloves and nutmeg until smooth. Pack into ramekins. Cover and refrigerate for at least 3 days or for up to 1 week.

TIPS

Substitute pecorino, aged Gouda, Gruyère, or almost any other hard or semi-hard cheese you like for the Parmesan.

Choose dry or sweet vermouth or sherry — it's up to you!

Parmesan Cheese Dip

1 cup	cubed Parmesan cheese	250 mL
1 cup	creamed cottage cheese	250 mL
2 tbsp	white vermouth or sherry	25 mL
1	clove garlic, smashed	1
¼ tsp	crumbled dried oregano	1 mL
¼ tsp	freshly ground black pepper	1 mL
Pinch	cayenne pepper	Pinch

1. In blender, on low speed, blend Parmesan until finely grated. Add cottage cheese, vermouth, garlic, oregano, black pepper and cayenne. Blend on high speed until smooth.

2. *Make ahead:* Cover and refrigerate for up to 1 week.

*Serve with fresh
sliced baguette or
baguette croûtes.*

TIP

Toast caraway seeds
in a small skillet
over medium-low
heat until fragrant
and seeds begin to
wiggle in pan, about
2 minutes.

Cheese and Onion Dip

¾ cup	cubed Swiss (Emmental) cheese	175 mL
¾ cup	cubed Gruyère cheese	175 mL
¼ cup	butter	50 mL
1	small onion, chopped	1
1	clove garlic, minced	1
¼ tsp	freshly ground black pepper	1 mL
⅓ cup	dry white wine	75 mL
2 tsp	Dijon mustard	10 mL
¼ cup	sour cream	50 mL
2 tsp	lightly toasted caraway seeds	10 mL

1. In blender, on low speed, blend Swiss and Gruyère cheeses until finely shredded. Set aside in the blender.

2. In a small skillet, heat butter over medium heat. Add onion, garlic and pepper; cook, stirring occasionally, until onions and garlic are golden, about 10 minutes. Add wine and mustard; bring to a boil.

3. Transfer to blender and purée on high speed. Pulse in sour cream until thoroughly mixed. Pulse in caraway seeds.

5. *Make ahead:* Cover and refrigerate for up to 1 week.

You're short on time and guests are arriving. The blender to the rescue with these quick dips!

Quick Cream Cheese Dips

Cream Cheese Dip Base

1	package (8 oz/250 g) cream cheese, cut into small cubes and softened	1
¼ cup	milk or sour cream (approx.)	50 mL
½ tsp	salt	2 mL
¼ tsp	freshly ground black pepper	1 mL

1. In blender, on low speed, blend cream cheese, milk, salt and pepper until smooth, adding more milk if necessary.

2. Blend with any of the following flavorings.

3. *Make ahead:* Cover and refrigerate for up to 3 days.

Smoked Fish Dip

6 oz	smoked salmon, mackerel, trout or other smoked fish (skinned)	175 g
4	red radishes, chopped	4
2 tbsp	minced red onion	25 mL
1 tsp	freshly squeezed lemon juice (or to taste)	5 mL

Anchovy Dip

1	can (1¾ oz/50 g) anchovies, drained	1
2 tbsp	chopped fresh parsley	25 mL
1 tbsp	capers, drained	15 mL

Blue Cheese Dip

½ cup	crumbled blue cheese (Danish, Roquefort, Gorgonzola, etc.)	125 mL
2 tbsp	sour cream	25 mL
1	green onion, chopped	1
	Chopped walnuts, for garnish (optional)	

Curry and Apple Dip

2 tsp	curry powder (see recipe, page 78) or curry paste	10 mL
1	apple, peeled, cored and chopped	1
1 tsp	liquid honey	5 mL
1 tsp	freshly squeezed lemon juice	5 mL

Onion and Garlic Dip

	1 onion, chopped, and 4 cloves garlic, chopped, lightly browned in 2 tbsp (25 mL) vegetable oil	
2 tbsp	chopped fresh chives	25 mL

Olive and Garlic Dip

1/3 cup	pitted olives	75 mL
1	clove garlic, smashed	1
2 tbsp	chopped fresh parsley or basil	25 mL
2 tsp	freshly squeezed lemon juice	10 mL

Tuna Dip

1	can (6.5 oz/184 g) tuna, drained	1
2 tbsp	chopped sweet onion	25 mL
1 tsp	freshly squeezed lemon juice (or to taste)	5 mL
1/2 tsp	Worcestershire sauce	2 mL

Fruit and Nut Dip

1/4 cup	chopped apple or pear	50 mL
1/4 cup	walnuts or pecans	50 mL
1/4 cup	chopped celery	50 mL
1/4 cup	golden raisins	50 mL
1 tsp	freshly squeezed lemon juice	5 mL

MAKES ABOUT
1½ CUPS (375 ML)

Serve as a dip with warmed or grilled pita, or spread on toast triangles as an hors d'oeuvre.

TIP

For a firmer cheese, drain for the full 2 days. Form cheese into small balls and place on a paper towel–lined tray. Refrigerate for 1 day. Store cheese balls in a jar filled with olive oil at room temperature for up to 1 week or in the refrigerator for up to 1 month.

Herbed Yogurt Cheese

1	large container (1½ lb/750 g) Balkan-style yogurt	1
½ cup	loosely packed mint or basil leaves (or 1 tbsp/15 mL chopped fresh thyme leaves)	125 mL
¼ tsp	salt (approx.)	1 mL
3 tbsp	extra-virgin olive oil	45 mL

1. In blender, on low speed, blend half the yogurt, mint and salt until mint is very finely chopped. Mix with remaining yogurt.

2. Line a sieve with cheesecloth or paper towels. Scrape yogurt mixture into sieve and place over a bowl. Refrigerate for 1 to 2 days, stirring yogurt mixture twice. Discard whey.

3. Scrape into a shallow serving bowl and check if additional salt is needed.

4. *Make ahead:* Cover and refrigerate for up to 3 days. To serve, drizzle top with olive oil.

MAKES ABOUT
1 CUP (250 ML)

Wonderful with fresh-cut veggies or potato chips.

Tarragon Mustard Dip

½ cup	mayonnaise (store-bought or see recipe, page 54)	125 mL
½ cup	sour cream (regular or light)	125 mL
2 tbsp	chopped fresh parsley or basil	25 mL
1 tbsp	white wine vinegar	15 mL
1 tbsp	tarragon mustard	15 mL
1 tsp	dried tarragon	5 mL
¼ tsp	salt	1 mL
¼ tsp	freshly ground black pepper	1 mL

1. In blender, on low speed, blend mayonnaise, sour cream, parsley, vinegar, mustard, tarragon, salt and black pepper until smooth.

2. *Make ahead:* Cover and refrigerate for up to 1 week.

This dip should be blended until absolutely smooth. The lemon flavor is intense.

TIP

You can substitute aged provolone, Parmesan or pecorino cheese for the Asiago as desired.

Lemony Eggplant Dip

● *Preheat oven to 400°F (200°C)*
● *Roasting pan*

2	Italian eggplants	2
1	lemon	1
2	cloves garlic, smashed	2
⅓ cup	extra-virgin olive oil	75 mL
⅓ cup	grated Asiago cheese	75 mL
¾ tsp	salt	4 mL
¼ tsp	freshly ground black pepper	1 mL
Pinch	cayenne pepper	Pinch

1. Place eggplant in a roasting pan and roast in preheated oven until flesh is soft when tested with fork, about 45 minutes. Let cool, then peel and scoop out flesh. Place in blender.

2. Meanwhile, with a vegetable peeler or zester remove yellow zest from lemon and add to blender. Peel off white pith and discard. Seed and chop flesh and add to blender with zest. Add garlic, oil, cheese, salt, pepper and cayenne; blend on high speed until smooth. Add eggplant and blend on low speed until smooth.

3. *Make ahead:* Cover and refrigerate for up to 3 days.

Avocado Dip

**MAKES ABOUT
1¼ CUPS (300 ML)**

This is another quick and easy crowd-pleasing dip. Unlike guacamole, which requires mashing by hand with a fork to get the proper texture, this avocado dip should be smooth and fluffy.

1	avocado	1
3	green onions, white part only, chopped	3
1	clove garlic, smashed	1
¼ cup	extra-virgin olive oil	50 mL
3 tbsp	freshly squeezed lemon juice	45 mL
½ tsp	salt	2 mL
¼ tsp	freshly ground black pepper	1 mL
¼ tsp	Mexican green hot pepper sauce or other hot pepper sauce	1 mL

1. Halve and pit avocado and scoop out flesh into blender. Add onions, garlic, oil, lemon juice, salt, pepper and hot pepper sauce; blend on low speed until smooth and fluffy.

Roasted Pepper Dip

**MAKES ABOUT
1⅓ CUPS (325 ML)**

The anchovies add an irreplaceable depth of flavor that is not at all fishy to this incredibly simple but delicious dip. Serve with warm bread or crudités.

- Preheat broiler
- Baking sheet

2	red bell peppers	2
½ cup	mayonnaise (store-bought or see recipe, page 54)	125 mL
¼ cup	sour cream	50 mL
2	anchovy fillets, rinsed and dried	2
1	clove garlic, smashed	1
1 tbsp	chopped fresh tarragon (or ½ tsp/2 mL dried)	15 mL

1. Quarter and seed peppers. Place skin side up on baking sheet and broil until skins are blackened. Let cool. Using fingers, slip off skins.

2. In blender, on high speed, purée seeded peeled peppers, mayonnaise, sour cream, anchovies, garlic and tarragon.

3. *Make ahead:* Cover and refrigerate for up to 3 days.

This dip is most flavorful if you cook and purée your own pumpkin or other winter squash, but in a pinch you can use canned pumpkin purée.

Curried Pumpkin Dip

2 tbsp	vegetable oil	25 mL
3	cloves garlic, minced	3
1	onion, chopped	1
1 tbsp	minced fresh gingerroot	15 mL
1 tsp	ground cumin	5 mL
1/2 tsp	ground coriander	2 mL
1/4 tsp	salt	1 mL
1/4 tsp	turmeric	1 mL
1/4 tsp	cayenne pepper	1 mL
Pinch	ground cloves	Pinch
1 cup	pumpkin or squash purée	250 mL
1/2 cup	cooked chickpeas (or drained, rinsed canned)	125 mL
1/2 cup	plain yogurt	125 mL
2 tbsp	freshly squeezed lemon juice	25 mL
2 tbsp	water	25 mL
1/4 cup	chopped fresh coriander	50 mL

1. In a skillet, heat oil over medium heat. Add garlic, onion, ginger, cumin, coriander, salt, turmeric, cayenne and cloves; cook, stirring, until onions are golden, about 6 minutes.

2. Transfer to blender and add pumpkin purée, chickpeas, yogurt, lemon juice, water and coriander. Blend on low speed, scraping down sides of blender as necessary, until smooth.

3. *Make ahead:* Cover and refrigerate for up to 3 days.

This dip is terrific with vegetable crudités and grilled pitas.

Roasted Garlic Dip

● *Preheat oven to 325°F (160°C)*

4	heads garlic	4
¼ cup	extra-virgin olive oil, divided	50 mL
1 cup	cold water	250 mL
3 cups	crustless white bread cubes	750 mL
⅓ cup	sour cream	75 mL
2 tsp	minced fresh sage (or ½ tsp/2 mL dried crumbled sage)	10 mL
¼ tsp	salt	1 mL
¼ tsp	freshly ground black pepper	1 mL

1. Cut top third off garlic heads. Place garlic cut side up on a large square of heavy-duty foil. Drizzle 2 tbsp (25 mL) of the olive oil over top, bring sides of foil up and seal to make package. Bake in center of preheated oven until garlic is very tender, about 1 hour. Let cool.

2. In a large bowl, drizzle cold water over bread cubes, tossing to moisten; squeeze out excess liquid.

3. In blender, combine bread, sour cream, remaining 2 tbsp (25 mL) oil, sage, salt and pepper. Squeeze garlic cloves out of skins into blender. Blend on low speed, scraping down sides of blender as necessary, until very smooth.

4. *Make ahead:* Cover and refrigerate for up to 1 day. Bring to room temperature before serving.

*It may sound unusual,
but this light
orange dip is sweet,
savory and delicious.
Serve with warmed
pita triangles.*

Roasted Carrot and Parsnip Dip

- Preheat oven to 425°F (220°C)
- Large rimmed baking sheet

5	carrots, peeled (about 12 oz/375 g)	5
5	parsnips, peeled (about 12 oz/375 g)	5
10	cloves garlic, peeled	10
2 tbsp	vegetable oil	25 mL
1/2 cup	mayonnaise (store-bought or see recipe, page 54)	125 mL
1/4 cup	sour cream	50 mL
1/4 cup	water	50 mL
1 tbsp	chopped fresh tarragon (or 1/2 tsp/2 mL dried)	15 mL
1 tbsp	tarragon-flavored vinegar	15 mL
Pinch	granulated sugar	Pinch
Pinch	salt	Pinch
Pinch	freshly ground black pepper	Pinch

1. Slice carrots and parsnips lengthwise into 1/2-inch (1 cm) thick slices. In a large bowl, toss carrots, parsnips, garlic and oil. Scrape onto baking sheet. Roast in bottom third of preheated oven until garlic is tender, about 20 minutes. Remove garlic. Turn carrots and parsnips over and continue roasting for 10 to 15 minutes, or until tender and browned.

2. In blender, on high speed, purée carrots, parsnips, garlic, mayonnaise, sour cream, water, tarragon, vinegar, sugar, salt and pepper. Transfer to a serving dish and let cool.

3. *Make ahead:* Cover and refrigerate for up to 4 days.

This is wonderful as a thin spread on a roasted vegetable sandwich or as a dip for vegetables or bread sticks.

Mushroom Dip

1	package (½ oz/14 g) dried shiitake mushrooms	1
½ cup	warm water	125 mL
2 tbsp	extra-virgin olive oil	25 mL
4	cloves garlic, minced	4
1	onion, chopped	1
3 cups	sliced mushrooms	750 mL
¼ tsp	salt	1 mL
¼ tsp	freshly ground black pepper	1 mL
2 tbsp	brandy	25 mL
½ cup	mayonnaise (store-bought or see recipe, page 54)	125 mL
¼ cup	chopped fresh flat-leaf parsley	50 mL
¼ cup	softened cream cheese (about 2 oz/60 g)	50 mL
2 tsp	chopped fresh thyme	10 mL
1 tsp	wine vinegar	5 mL

1. In a small bowl, soak shiitake mushrooms in warm water until soft, about 30 minutes. Drain, reserving liquid, remove stems and discard (or save for stock pot). Chop caps finely.

2. In a skillet, heat oil over medium-high heat. Add garlic, onion, mushrooms, shiitake caps, salt and pepper; cook, stirring, until liquid is evaporated and mixture is beginning to turn golden, about 10 minutes. Pour in reserved soaking liquid and brandy, bring to a boil and scrape up any brown bits with a spoon.

3. Transfer to blender and add mayonnaise, parsley, cream cheese, thyme and vinegar; blend on low speed until smooth.

4. *Make ahead:* Cover and refrigerate for up to 3 days.

Twenty years ago, few North Americans had heard of tapenade. Now it's a standard ingredient and is sold in jars everywhere. But it's so easy to make and tastes better homemade — and you can choose the variety of olive you want to use. It's good as a dip, a spread for sandwiches or a pizza topping.

Tapenade

6	anchovy fillets	6
1	clove garlic, smashed	1
½ cup	pitted black olives	125 mL
⅓ cup	extra-virgin olive oil	75 mL
¼ cup	loosely packed fresh basil leaves	50 mL
3 tbsp	freshly squeezed lemon juice	45 mL
4 tsp	drained capers	20 mL
¼ tsp	freshly ground black pepper	1 mL

1. Rinse anchovies under cold water. Place in blender and add garlic, olives, oil, basil, lemon juice, capers and pepper. Blend on high speed for 20 to 30 seconds, or until fairly smooth.

2. *Make ahead:* Cover and refrigerate for up to 2 weeks.

Serve this unusual, tasty dip with warmed pita triangles.

Walnut and Olive Dip

1	clove garlic, minced	1
2 cups	kalamata olives, pitted	500 mL
⅔ cup	toasted walnuts, finely chopped, divided	150 mL
3 tbsp	walnut oil or extra-virgin olive oil	45 mL
2 tsp	minced fresh oregano (or ½ tsp/2 mL dried)	10 mL
Pinch	freshly ground black pepper	Pinch
3 tbsp	water (approx.)	45 mL

1. In blender, on high speed, purée garlic, olives, ⅓ cup (75 mL) of the walnuts, oil, oregano and pepper. With motor running, add water 1 tbsp (15 mL) at a time, scraping down sides of blender as necessary, until a smooth, thin paste forms.

2. Scrape into a serving bowl and stir in the remaining ⅓ cup (75 mL) walnuts.

3. *Make ahead:* Cover and refrigerate for up to 2 days. Bring to room temperature before serving.

*Hummus is a
popular chickpea dip
for pita bread and
vegetable crudités.*

TIP

You can make the
same dip with fava
beans or white
kidney beans.

Quick Hummus

1	can (19 oz/540 mL) chickpeas, drained and rinsed	1
1	clove garlic, smashed	1
1/3 cup	freshly squeezed lemon juice	75 mL
1/3 cup	extra-virgin olive oil	75 mL
1/2 tsp	salt	2 mL
1/4 tsp	cayenne pepper	1 mL
1/4 tsp	ground cumin	1 mL
1/3 cup	tahini paste	75 mL

Garnish

2 tbsp	chopped fresh cilantro or parsley	25 mL
1/4 tsp	sweet paprika	1 mL
1 tbsp	extra-virgin olive oil	15 mL
6	black olives	6

1. In blender, on high speed, purée chickpeas, garlic, lemon juice, oil, salt, cayenne and cumin. Reduce speed to low, add Tahini Paste and blend until fully incorporated, scraping down sides as necessary.

2. *Make ahead:* Cover and refrigerate for up to 3 days. To serve, sprinkle with cilantro and paprika and drizzle with oil. Scatter olives over top.

Tahini Dip

⅔ cup	tahini paste	150 mL
1	clove garlic, smashed	1
½ tsp	salt	2 mL
½ tsp	sweet paprika	2 mL
¼ tsp	cayenne pepper	1 mL
¼ tsp	ground cumin	1 mL
⅓ cup	freshly squeezed lemon juice	75 mL
½ cup	water (approx.)	125 mL

Garnish

2 tbsp	minced fresh parsley	25 mL
¼ tsp	paprika	1 mL

1. In blender, on low speed, blend tahini paste, garlic, salt, paprika, cayenne and cumin. With motor running, through hole in top, gradually pour in lemon juice and just enough water until desired consistency.

2. *Make ahead:* Cover and refrigerate for up to 1 week. To serve, sprinkle with parsley and paprika.

TIP

For a chunky peanut butter, reserve ¼ cup (50 mL) of the peanuts and add them at the end of blending.

Natural Peanut Butter

1½ cups	roasted salted or unsalted peanuts	375 mL
1 tbsp	peanut oil, sesame oil or vegetable oil	15 mL
2 tsp	maple syrup or liquid honey (optional)	10 mL

1. In blender, on high speed, purée peanuts, oil and maple syrup (if using), scraping down sides as necessary.

2. Store in the refrigerator for up to 3 months.

Another easy dip for harried entertainers, this can be assembled in a few minutes and will prove to be the hit of the hors d'oeuvres table. Serve with rye or whole wheat croûtes.

Quick and Easy Smoked Fish Dip

12 oz	smoked mackerel or trout fillets, skinned	375 g
½ cup	sour cream	125 mL
½ cup	dry cottage cheese	125 mL
2 tbsp	freshly squeezed lemon juice	25 mL
¼ tsp	sweet paprika	1 mL
¼ tsp	salt	1 mL
¼ tsp	freshly ground black pepper	1 mL
Pinch	cayenne pepper	Pinch
2 tbsp	minced fresh chives or parsley	25 mL

1. Flake fish and place in blender. Add sour cream, cottage cheese, lemon juice, paprika, salt, pepper and cayenne; blend on low speed until smooth. Pulse in chives.

2. *Make ahead:* Cover and refrigerate for up to 1 day.

Serve this thick, savory dip, lightly flavored with smoked trout, with endive spears or crudités.

Smoked Trout and Pepper Dip

1 cup	sour cream	250 mL
½ cup	cream cheese, softened (about 4 oz/125 g)	125 mL
2 tsp	freshly squeezed lemon juice	10 mL
2 oz	smoked trout or salmon (skinned)	60 g
1 tsp	cracked mixed peppercorns	5 mL
1 tbsp	minced fresh chives	15 mL

1. In blender, on high speed, purée sour cream, cream cheese and lemon juice, scraping down sides as necessary. Add trout and pulse until combined.

2. Scrape into a serving bowl. Stir in peppercorns and sprinkle with chives.

3. *Make ahead:* Cover and refrigerate for up to 3 days.

For another quick dip, all you need is 2 cans of boneless sardines and a few common pantry items.

TIP

For a smoky flavor, use smoked sprats instead of sardines, but you'll have to bone them yourself.

Sardine Dip

2	cans (each 4.4 oz/125 g) boneless sardines, drained	2
1	package (8 oz/250 g) cream cheese, cut in cubes and softened	1
½ cup	lightly packed fresh parsley leaves	125 mL
¼ cup	grated sweet onion	50 mL
3 tbsp	freshly squeezed lemon juice or lime juice	45 mL
2 tbsp	extra-virgin olive oil	25 mL
½ tsp	salt	2 mL
Dash	hot pepper sauce	Dash
	Milk	

1. In blender, on low speed, blend sardines, cream cheese, parsley, onion, lemon juice, olive oil, salt and hot pepper sauce until smooth, scraping down sides and adding milk as necessary to make a good dipping consistency.

2. *Make ahead:* Cover and refrigerate for up to 3 days.

This English treat, irresistible for lovers of smoked fish, is a wonderful treat for the buffet table or as an hors d'oeuvre. Serve with Melba toast or pumpernickel rounds.

Kipper Pâté

12 oz	kipper fillets	375 g
2 tbsp	butter	25 mL
1	clove garlic, minced	1
2 tbsp	minced onion	25 mL
2 tbsp	whipping (35%) cream	25 mL
2 tbsp	freshly squeezed lemon juice	25 mL
1 tbsp	brandy	15 mL
Dash	hot pepper sauce	Dash

1. Poach kippers in barely simmering water, about 4 minutes. Drain. Remove skin and bones and place flesh in blender.

2. In a small skillet, melt butter over medium heat. Add garlic and onion; cook, stirring, for 4 minutes, until soft.

3. Transfer to blender and add whipping cream, lemon juice, brandy and hot pepper sauce. Blend on low speed until smooth.

Brandade

1 lb	boneless skinless salt cod	500 g
2	cloves garlic, smashed	2
1	large potato, boiled and coarsely chopped	1
1 cup	extra-virgin olive oil, divided	250 mL
¾ cup	milk, divided	175 mL
3 tbsp	freshly squeezed lemon juice	45 mL
¼ tsp	freshly grated nutmeg	1 mL
¼ tsp	freshly ground white pepper	1 mL
	Salt	

1. Soak cod overnight (or for up to 24 hours) in several changes of cold water. Taste to see if cod is sufficiently desalted. Drain.

2. In a medium saucepan, cover cod with cold water; heat over high heat until simmering. Remove from heat and let cool. Drain and flake fish into blender.

3. Add garlic, potato, and half of each of the oil and the milk. Purée on low speed, about 1 minute. Scrape down sides and blend on high for 2 minutes, until quite sticky.

4. With blender on low speed, very gradually add remaining milk in a slow stream through hole in top, for about 3 minutes, periodically scraping down sides and stirring as necessary. Then gradually add remaining oil in a thin stream through hole in top, for 3 to 4 minutes, periodically scraping down sides and stirring as necessary.

5. Blend for a further 2 minutes on high until fluffy and light-colored. On low speed, add lemon juice, nutmeg and pepper. Add salt to taste.

6. Scrape into a clean saucepan and cook over low heat, stirring constantly, for 5 to 7 minutes, or until warm but not simmering.

**MAKES ABOUT
1¾ CUPS (425 ML)**

*This southern French
dip for vegetable
crudités is usually
served in a ceramic
dish over a tea light
flame to keep it warm.
It can be spooned over
cold leftover roast
pork or veal, or boiled
beef or chicken.*

TIP

Two 1¾ oz (50 g)
cans of anchovies
yield about
24 anchovy fillets.

Bagna Cauda

24	anchovy fillets	24
4	thick slices white bread, crusts removed	4
3	cloves garlic, smashed	3
½ tsp	freshly ground black pepper	2 mL
1 cup	extra-virgin olive oil	250 mL
2 tbsp	butter	25 mL

1. Soak anchovies in water for 20 minutes. Drain and rinse under cold water.

2. Sprinkle bread with water until soft. Squeeze out excess water and tear into pieces.

3. Place anchovies and bread in blender and add garlic and pepper. On low speed, blend into a paste, scraping down sides as necessary. With motor running, add oil through hole in top in a thin stream and blend until smooth.

4. In a small saucepan, melt butter over low heat. Scrape anchovy sauce into pan and heat through, stirring constantly, for about 7 minutes.

**MAKES ABOUT
½ CUP (125 ML)**

TIP

For tasty tapas, spread
thinly over toasted
bread triangles and
top with capers,
roasted red pepper,
minced red onion
and finely chopped
hard-cooked egg, or
fresh basil chiffonade.

Anchovy Spread

5	cloves garlic	5
24	anchovy fillets (see tip, above)	24
¼ cup	pasteurized liquid whole egg	50 mL
½ tsp	freshly ground black pepper	2 mL
¼ cup	extra virgin olive oil	50 mL
2 tbsp	minced parsley	25 mL

1. In small saucepan of boiling water, poach garlic for 3 minutes. Drain and place in blender.

2. Rinse anchovies under cold water, drain and place in blender with egg yolks and pepper. Purée on low speed, about 1 minute. On high speed, gradually add oil in thin stream through top until incorporated and emulsified. Stir in parsley.

**MAKES ABOUT
2 CUPS (500 ML)**

*A lovely English pâté
for chicken lovers,
this is actually much
lighter than you would
imagine. Serve with
crackers or bread, or
use as a filling for tea
sandwiches, with thin
slices of cucumber or
watercress sprigs.*

Chicken Pâté

1	bunch green onions	1
6	strips bacon, sliced	6
4	boneless skinless chicken thighs, chopped (about 12 oz/375 g)	4
2 tbsp	dry sherry	25 mL
½ cup	cream cheese, cubed (about 4 oz/125 g)	125 mL
2 tbsp	sour cream	25 mL
2 tbsp	chopped fresh parsley	25 mL

1. Separate white and green parts of onions. Chop white parts and thinly slice green parts.

2. In a skillet, over medium heat, cook bacon, stirring, until lightly browned, about 5 minutes. Add white part of onions and chicken; cook, stirring often, until chicken is no longer pink inside, about 4 minutes. Add sherry and cook, stirring, for 30 seconds, scraping up brown bits stuck to pan.

3. Transfer to blender and add cream cheese, sour cream and parsley. Blend on low speed until smooth. Pulse in green part of onions.

4. *Make ahead:* Cover and refrigerate for up to 1 day.

My good friend Angela Boyd gave us this excellent recipe. Serve with baguette croûtes.

Chicken Liver Pâté

- Preheat oven to 325°F (160°C)
- 9- by 5-inch (2 L) loaf pan
- Roasting pan

2 lbs	chicken livers	1 kg
1/3 cup	butter	75 mL
3	cloves garlic, minced	3
3	eggs	3
1/3 cup	all-purpose flour	75 mL
2 tbsp	brandy, sherry or port	25 mL
1 tsp	salt	5 mL
1/4 tsp	ground allspice	1 mL
1/4 tsp	ground ginger	1 mL
1/4 tsp	ground nutmeg	1 mL
1/4 tsp	freshly ground black pepper	1 mL

1. Separate lobes of liver, discarding any connective tissue and sinew. Cut each larger lobe in half.

2. In a skillet, melt butter over medium heat. Add garlic and cook, stirring, until fragrant, about 30 seconds. Add liver and cook, stirring, until browned all over but centers are still pink, about 4 minutes.

3. Transfer to blender and add eggs, flour, brandy, salt, allspice, ginger, nutmeg and pepper. Blend on low speed, scraping down sides as necessary, until smooth.

4. Scrape into loaf pan and cover with foil. Place in roasting pan and pour in 2 inches (5 cm) boiling water. Bake in preheated oven for 2 hours, until meat thermometer inserted in center registers 180°F (85°C). Uncover and let cool completely in pan on a rack.

5. Cover pâté with plastic wrap and place a piece of cardboard cut to fit inside loaf pan on top of plastic. Weigh down with weights (canned goods are convenient) and refrigerate for at least 4 hours or for up to 2 days. Bring to room temperature before serving.

*If you don't have time
to make a traditional
chicken liver pâté,
make this quick and
delicious spread.*

TIP

You can buy rendered
chicken fat at Jewish
grocers or make your
own: In a medium
saucepan, combine
2 cups (500 mL)
chopped chicken fat
with ¼ cup (50 mL)
water. Over low
heat, cook until fat
cracklings are brown
and fat is rendered,
about 30 minutes. If
desired, add ½ cup
(125 mL) chopped
onion with fat.

Quick Chicken Liver and Mushroom Spread

8 oz	chicken livers	250 g
12	white mushrooms	12
½	white onion, chopped	½
	Water	
½ cup	butter, softened, or rendered chicken fat	125 mL
1 tbsp	dry sherry	15 mL
½ tsp	salt	2 mL
¼ tsp	freshly ground black pepper	1 mL

1. Trim any connective tissue and sinew from livers.

2. In a medium saucepan, combine livers, mushrooms and onion and add enough water to barely cover. Bring to a simmer over high heat. Reduce heat to low and simmer until livers are just pink in center, about 15 minutes. Drain in colander.

3. Transfer to blender and add butter, sherry, salt and pepper; blend on low speed, scraping down sides as necessary, until smooth.

4. *Make ahead:* Cover and refrigerate for up to 1 day. Bring to room temperature before serving.

Salad Dressings

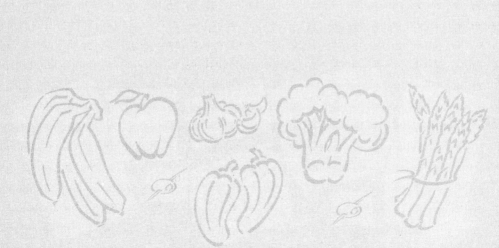

*Sesame oil and
seeds make this
raspberry dressing
an unusual treat.*

Raspberry Dressing

2	cloves garlic	2
1/3 cup	fresh or frozen raspberries	75 mL
1/4 cup	peanut or vegetable oil	50 mL
1/4 cup	raspberry-flavored vinegar	50 mL
2 tbsp	sesame oil	25 mL
2 tbsp	balsamic vinegar	25 mL
2 tsp	Dijon mustard	10 mL
1/4 tsp	salt	1 mL
1/4 tsp	freshly ground black pepper	1 mL
2 tbsp	toasted sesame seeds	25 mL

1. In blender, on high speed, purée garlic, raspberries, peanut oil, raspberry-flavored vinegar, sesame oil, balsamic vinegar, mustard, salt and pepper. Strain through a fine sieve into a bowl or jar. Add sesame seeds. Shake before using.

2. *Make ahead:* Cover and refrigerate for up to 1 week.

*This sweet-and-sour
dressing can be
drizzled over blanched
and chilled cauliflower
or other vegetables,
or over crispy
lettuce salad.*

Poppy Seed Dressing

1	small clove garlic, smashed	1
1/4	sweet onion, chopped	1/4
1/3 cup	liquid honey	75 mL
1/4 cup	freshly squeezed lemon juice	50 mL
2 tbsp	cider vinegar or white wine vinegar	25 mL
2 tsp	Dijon mustard	10 mL
1/2 tsp	salt	2 mL
1/4 tsp	hot pepper sauce	1 mL
2 tbsp	poppy seeds	25 mL
1 cup	extra-virgin olive oil	250 mL

1. In blender, on low speed, blend garlic, onion, honey, lemon juice, vinegar, mustard, salt and hot pepper sauce until onion and garlic are finely chopped. Add poppy seeds. With motor running, through hole in top, gradually pour in oil in a thin stream until blended.

2. *Make ahead:* Cover and refrigerate for up to 1 week.

*Try this dressing
drizzled over sliced
cucumber, tomato and
sweet onion.*

TIP

For a thinner dressing,
add a little water.

Avocado Dressing

1	avocado, peeled and chopped	1
1	small clove garlic, smashed	1
½ cup	buttermilk or yogurt	125 mL
2 tbsp	extra-virgin olive oil	25 mL
2 tbsp	freshly squeezed lemon juice	25 mL
1 tbsp	white wine vinegar	15 mL
½ tsp	salt	2 mL
¼ tsp	freshly ground black pepper	1 mL
Pinch	ground cumin	Pinch
Dash	hot pepper sauce	Dash

1. In blender, on low speed, purée avocado, garlic, buttermilk, oil, lemon juice, vinegar, salt, pepper, cumin and hot pepper sauce.

2. *Make ahead:* Cover and refrigerate for up to 3 days.

*This is a refreshing
dressing for a salad
of lettuce and sliced
radishes, as well as
a sauce for poached
salmon, hot or cold.*

TIP

Instead of the cilantro,
try 2 tsp (10 mL)
fresh dill.

Cucumber Dressing

⅔ cup	sour cream or yogurt	150 mL
2 tbsp	freshly squeezed lemon juice	25 mL
¼ tsp	salt	1 mL
¼ tsp	freshly ground black pepper	1 mL
¼ tsp	granulated sugar	1 mL
Pinch	cayenne pepper or paprika	Pinch
1	field cucumber (or ½ English cucumber), peeled, seeded and chopped	1
2 tbsp	chopped fresh cilantro (or 2 tsp/10 mL chopped fresh dill)	25 mL
1 tbsp	chopped chives or green onions	15 mL

1. In blender, on high speed, mix sour cream, lemon juice, salt, pepper, sugar and cayenne until thick. Add cucumber and blend on low speed until very finely chopped. Pulse in cilantro and chives.

2. *Make ahead:* Cover and refrigerate for up to 3 days.

The peppery flavor of watercress enhances this dressing, which is suitable for potato salad as well as mixed greens.

Watercress Dressing I

2	hard-cooked egg yolks	2
1 cup	lightly packed watercress, tough stems removed	250 mL
⅓ cup	extra-virgin olive oil	75 mL
2 tbsp	sherry vinegar or red wine vinegar	25 mL
¼ tsp	salt	1 mL
¼ tsp	freshly ground black pepper	1 mL
½ tsp	Dijon mustard	2 mL
¼ tsp	anchovy paste (optional)	1 mL

1. In blender, on low speed, blend egg yolks, watercress, oil, vinegar, salt, pepper, mustard and anchovy paste (if using), until smooth.

2. *Make ahead:* Cover and refrigerate for up to 3 days.

Use this dressing on cold blanched vegetables or cucumbers and mixed greens. It also is excellent for chicken, veal or ham salad.

Watercress Dressing II

2	hard-cooked eggs, quartered	2
½	clove garlic, smashed	½
⅓ cup	extra-virgin olive oil	75 mL
2 tbsp	freshly squeezed lemon juice	25 mL
4 tsp	wine vinegar	20 mL
½ tsp	salt	2 mL
Pinch	freshly ground black pepper	Pinch
1 cup	lightly packed watercress, tough stems removed	250 mL

1. In blender, on low speed, blend eggs, garlic, oil, lemon juice, vinegar, salt and pepper until smooth. Add watercress and pulse until finely chopped.

2. *Make ahead:* Cover and refrigerate for up to 3 days.

Garlic Dressing

*This dressing is
delicious on blanched
or steamed green or
wax beans or drizzled
over boiled potatoes.
Try it as a dip for warm
or cold vegetables, or
toss it with a salad of
boldly flavored mixed
greens. If you use
the egg yolk, you'll
have a thicker and
creamier dressing.*

*This recipe contains an
optional raw egg yolk.
If the food safety of
raw eggs is a concern
for you, omit the egg
yolk or use the
pasteurized liquid
whole egg instead.*

¼ cup	garlic cloves (unpeeled)	50 mL
1	egg yolk (or 2 tbsp/25 mL pasteurized liquid whole egg) (optional)	1
3 tbsp	sherry vinegar	45 mL
¼ tsp	salt	1 mL
¼ tsp	freshly ground black pepper	1 mL
Dash	hot pepper sauce	Dash
⅔ cup	extra-virgin olive oil	150 mL
¼ cup	chopped chives or minced green onions	50 mL

1. In a small saucepan of boiling water, cook garlic until tender, about 8 minutes. Drain and chill under cold water and slip off peels.

2. In blender, on high speed, purée blanched garlic, egg yolk (if using), vinegar, salt, pepper and hot pepper sauce. With motor running, through hole in top, gradually pour in oil in a thin stream until smooth. Pulse in chives.

3. *Make ahead:* Cover and refrigerate for up to 3 days.

Variation

Roasted Garlic Dressing: Substitute 2 heads of roasted garlic for the blanched garlic. To roast, cut off top ends of whole heads of garlic. Drizzle with oil and wrap in foil. Roast in a 400°F (200°C) toaster oven or oven until tender, 30 to 40 minutes. Squeeze cloves out of skins.

*Use this dressing in
the same way as the
version on page 37.
For a dressing for
boiled potatoes or
to use as a dip
for crudités,
add 2 hard-cooked
egg yolks along with
the garlic.*

Lightened-Up Garlic Dressing

¼ cup	garlic cloves (unpeeled)	50 mL
½ cup	buttermilk	125 mL
¼ cup	extra-virgin olive oil	50 mL
3 tbsp	sherry vinegar	45 mL
¼ tsp	salt	1 mL
¼ tsp	freshly ground black pepper	1 mL
¼ cup	chopped chives or minced green onions	50 mL

1. In a small saucepan of boiling water, cook garlic until tender, about 8 minutes. Drain and chill under cold water and slip off peels.

2. In blender, on high speed, purée blanched garlic, buttermilk, oil, vinegar, salt and pepper. Pulse in chives.

3. *Make ahead:* Cover and refrigerate for up to 3 days.

Variation

Lightened-Up Roasted Garlic Dressing: Substitute 2 heads of roasted garlic for the blanched garlic. To roast, cut off top ends of whole heads of garlic. Drizzle with oil and wrap in foil. Roast in a 400°F (200°C) toaster oven or oven until tender, 30 to 40 minutes. Squeeze cloves out of skins.

Drizzle this dressing over greens and top with goat cheese and toasted pine nuts.

Roasted Garlic and Rosemary Dressing

● *Preheat oven to 400°F (200°C)*

4	heads garlic	4
½ cup	extra-virgin olive oil, divided	125 mL
¼ cup	sherry or wine vinegar	50 mL
1 tsp	minced fresh rosemary	5 mL
2 tsp	grainy mustard	10 mL
¼ tsp	salt	1 mL
¼ tsp	freshly ground black pepper	1 mL
Pinch	granulated sugar	Pinch

1. Cut top third off garlic heads. Place garlic cut side up on a large square of heavy-duty foil and drizzle with 2 tbsp (25 mL) of the olive oil. Bring sides of foil up and seal to make package. Bake in center of preheated oven for 30 to 40 minutes, or until garlic is very tender. Let cool.

2. Squeeze garlic cloves out of skins into blender. Add remaining oil, vinegar, rosemary, mustard, salt, pepper and sugar and purée on high speed.

3. *Make ahead:* Cover and refrigerate for up to 3 days.

Top a salad of cucumber, bean sprouts and tender raw or blanched cabbage or iceberg lettuce with this piquant peanut dressing. For a more substantial salad, add some deep-fried cubes of tofu and/or hard-cooked eggs.

TIPS

To make tamarind juice, mix 1 tbsp (15 mL) tamarind paste with 3 tbsp (45 mL) water and strain out seeds and pulp.

Substitute 1 tsp (5 mL) shrimp paste for the fish sauce. In a dry skillet, over medium heat, fry shrimp paste, stirring often, until dry and roasted, about 4 minutes, before adding to blender with other ingredients.

Southeast Asian–Style Peanut Dressing

2	Thai bird chili peppers (or 1 hot pepper), chopped	2
1	clove garlic, chopped	1
¼ cup	natural crunchy peanut butter	50 mL
2 tbsp	tamarind juice (see tip, at left) or juice of 1 lime	25 mL
2 tsp	granulated sugar	10 mL
2 tsp	fish sauce	10 mL
2 tbsp	water (approx.)	25 mL

1. In blender, on low speed, blend chili peppers, garlic, peanut butter, tamarind juice, sugar and fish sauce, adding water as necessary to achieve desired consistency. Finish by puréeing on high speed if a very smooth sauce is desired.

2. *Make ahead:* Cover and refrigerate for up to 3 days. Bring to room temperature before using.

**MAKES ABOUT
2 CUPS (500 ML)**

Anybody who has been to Great Britain is familiar with salad cream, a sweet salad dressing that is as ubiquitous on table tops as ketchup is in North America. It's easy to buy prepared salad cream, but it's even easier, better tasting — and more economical — to make.

English Salad Cream

3 tbsp	all-purpose flour	45 mL
1¾ cup	milk	425 mL
3 tbsp	granulated sugar	45 mL
1 tbsp	Dijon mustard	15 mL
¼ tsp	celery salt	1 mL
¼ tsp	salt	1 mL
Pinch	freshly ground white pepper	Pinch
Pinch	cayenne pepper (optional)	Pinch
¼ cup	butter or margarine, melted (or vegetable oil)	50 mL
¼ cup	pasteurized liquid egg	50 mL
½ cup	cider vinegar	125 mL

1. Place flour in blender. With motor running on low speed, pour in milk through hole in top and blend until smooth. Add sugar, mustard, celery salt, salt, pepper and cayenne (if using) and blend until incorporated. Blend in butter.

2. Transfer to a saucepan and bring to a simmer over medium-low heat, stirring constantly; cook until thick and creamy. Remove from heat and whisk in egg.

3. Scrape into blender. With motor running on low speed, through hole in top, gradually pour in vinegar and blend until incorporated.

4. Store in the refrigerator for up to 1 month.

This classic sweet-and-sour North American dressing is similar to salad cream. It definitely belongs in the category of nostalgic recipes, and it's perfect for a "retro" salad of iceberg wedges, sliced cucumber and tomato. If you like sweet-and-sour dressings, try it on potato salad or coleslaw, or use it as a sandwich spread. Kids love it!

Nostalgic Sweet-and-Sour Dressing

¼ cup	pasteurized liquid egg	50 mL
¾ cup	sweetened condensed milk	175 mL
¼ cup	cider vinegar	50 mL
¼ cup	vegetable oil	50 mL
2 tbsp	freshly squeezed lemon juice	25 mL
2 tsp	Dijon mustard	10 mL
¼ tsp	salt	1 mL
¼ tsp	celery salt	1 mL
Pinch	freshly ground white pepper	Pinch
Dash	hot pepper sauce	Dash

1. In blender, on high speed, blend egg, condensed milk, vinegar, oil, lemon juice, mustard, salt, celery salt, pepper and hot pepper sauce until thick and creamy.

2. Store in the refrigerator for up to 1 month.

Try this delicious low-calorie salad dressing drizzled on hard-cooked eggs or pasta salad.

Buttermilk Dressing

2	green onions, chopped	2
1	small clove garlic, smashed	1
½ cup	buttermilk	125 mL
¼ cup	packed fresh parsley leaves	50 mL
2 tbsp	freshly squeezed lemon juice	25 mL
2 tbsp	extra-virgin olive oil	25 mL
1 tbsp	cider vinegar	15 mL
1 tsp	fresh tarragon leaves (or ½ tsp/2 mL dried)	5 mL
¼ tsp	salt	1 mL
Pinch	freshly ground white pepper	Pinch

1. In blender, on high speed, purée green onions, garlic, buttermilk, parsley, lemon juice, oil, vinegar, tarragon, salt and pepper.

2. *Make ahead:* Cover and refrigerate for up to 3 days.

Blue Cheese Dressing

Use this dressing for salads of bitter greens, such as curly endive, escarole or frisée lettuce, or as a dip for vegetable crudités.

TIP

For a thinner dressing, stir in buttermilk or milk to desired consistency.

1	small clove garlic, smashed	1
2/3 cup	crumbled blue cheese	150 mL
1/2 cup	sour cream	125 mL
1/3 cup	olive oil or vegetable oil	75 mL
1 tbsp	cider vinegar or wine vinegar	15 mL
2 tsp	Dijon mustard or prepared horseradish	10 mL
1/2 tsp	freshly ground black pepper	2 mL
Pinch	salt	Pinch

1. In blender, on high speed, purée garlic, blue cheese, sour cream, oil, vinegar, mustard, pepper and salt.

2. *Make ahead:* Cover and refrigerate for up to 1 week.

Thousand Island Dressing

This is my favorite of many variations of this classic nostalgic dressing.

8	pimento-stuffed green olives	8
1	hard-cooked egg yolk (optional)	1
1/4 cup	chopped green bell pepper	50 mL
1 cup	mayonnaise (store-bought or see recipe, page 54)	250 mL
1/4 cup	chili sauce or ketchup	50 mL
2 tbsp	chopped watercress leaves (optional)	25 mL
2 tbsp	chopped green onion	25 mL
2 tbsp	chopped fresh chives	25 mL
1 tbsp	chopped fresh parsley	15 mL
1 tbsp	cider vinegar	15 mL
3/4 tsp	granulated sugar	4 mL

1. In blender, on low speed, blend olives, egg yolk (if using), green pepper, mayonnaise, chili sauce, watercress, green onion, chives, parsley, vinegar and sugar, scraping down sides as necessary, until almost smooth.

2. *Make ahead:* Cover and refrigerate for up to 1 week.

Particularly good with spinach salad.

Creamy Honey-Mustard Dressing

¼ cup	rice vinegar or cider vinegar	50 mL
2 tbsp	hot honey mustard (store-bought or see recipe, page 52)	25 mL
1 tsp	dried thyme	5 mL
¾ cup	extra-virgin olive oil	175 mL
¼ tsp	salt	1 mL
¼ tsp	freshly ground black pepper	1 mL

1. In blender, on low speed, combine vinegar, mustard and thyme. With motor running, though hole in top, gradually pour in oil and blend until thick and smooth, scraping sides if necessary. Blend in salt and pepper.

2. *Make ahead:* Cover and refrigerate for up to 1 week.

Russian Dressing

1	hard-cooked egg, chopped	1
1	ripe tomato, peeled, seeded and quartered (or 1 canned tomato, seeded and quartered)	1
1 cup	mayonnaise (store-bought or see recipe, page 54)	250 mL
1 tbsp	chopped fresh parsley	15 mL
1 tbsp	chopped fresh dill	15 mL
1 tbsp	prepared horseradish	15 mL
1 tbsp	chopped dill pickle	15 mL
2 tsp	minced onion	10 mL

1. In blender, on low speed, blend egg, tomato, mayonnaise, parsley, dill, horseradish, pickle and onion until very finely chopped.

2. *Make ahead:* Cover and refrigerate for up to 3 days.

Drizzle this dressing over iceberg lettuce and tomato wedges for a lightened-up retro salad. For a lunch plate, add slices of hard-cooked egg, cubes of Swiss cheese and smoked ham, and serve with buttered pumpernickel bread.

Lightened-Up Russian Dressing

1	hard-cooked egg, quartered	1
1	ripe tomato, peeled, seeded and halved	1
½ cup	buttermilk	125 mL
2 tbsp	vegetable oil	25 mL
2 tbsp	cider vinegar or wine vinegar	25 mL
1 tbsp	prepared horseradish	15 mL
2	1-inch (2.5 cm) pieces dill pickle	2
1 tbsp	drained capers	15 mL
¼ cup	chopped chives	50 mL
¼ cup	chopped fresh parsley	50 mL
1 tbsp	chopped fresh dill	15 mL

1. In blender, on high speed, purée egg, tomato, buttermilk, oil, vinegar and horseradish. Add pickle and capers and pulse until chopped. Pulse in chives, parsley and dill.

2. *Make ahead:* Cover and refrigerate for up to 3 days.

Caesar Salad Dressing

North America's favorite salad, Caesar salad depends on a tasty combination of anchovies, Parmesan cheese, lemon juice, garlic and vinaigrette. Grate your own Italian Parmigiano-Reggiano or Grana Padano for best results, and, of course, use freshly ground black pepper.

4	anchovy fillets	4
3	cloves garlic, smashed	3
1/4 cup	pasteurized liquid egg	50 mL
1/4 cup	freshly squeezed lemon juice	50 mL
2 tbsp	red wine vinegar	25 mL
1/2 tsp	freshly ground black pepper	2 mL
Pinch	salt	Pinch
1/2 tsp	Worcestershire sauce	2 mL
Dash	hot pepper sauce	Dash
1 1/4 cup	extra-virgin olive oil	300 mL
1 cup	freshly grated Parmesan cheese	250 mL

TIPS

Makes enough dressing for 2 large heads of romaine lettuce. Each head of lettuce will make 4 to 6 salad servings, or 3 lunch or dinner servings.

The dressing will become quite thick after refrigeration. If your lettuce is very dry, thin dressing with 1 to 2 tbsp (15 to 25 mL) warm water.

1. In blender, on low speed, blend anchovies, garlic, egg, lemon juice, vinegar, pepper, salt, Worcestershire sauce and hot pepper sauce until smooth and creamy.

2. With motor running, though hole in top, gradually pour in oil in a very thin stream and blend until smooth. Add cheese and blend until incorporated.

3. *Make ahead:* Cover and refrigerate for up to 3 days.

Condiments, Sauces and Marinades

Classic Tomato Ketchup

Once you have tasted homemade ketchup, you will never want to use commercial ketchup again. This is, of course, an essential ingredient for hamburgers, grilled cheese sandwiches and Beer-Battered Onion Rings (see recipe, page 170).

TIP

You can substitute 3 lbs (1.5 kg) fresh tomatoes for the canned. Blanch in boiling water until skins begin to peel away, about 15 seconds. With a slotted spoon, remove tomatoes and place in ice water. With a paring knife, peel off skin, then scrape out seeds with a spoon.

3	cloves garlic, minced	3
1	small onion, chopped	1
1	stalk celery, chopped	1
1	can (28 oz/796 mL) diced tomatoes, with juice	1
1	can (5½ oz/156 mL) tomato paste	1
⅔ cup	cider vinegar	150 mL
⅓ cup	granulated sugar	75 mL
1 tbsp	pickling spice	15 mL
1 tsp	celery seed	5 mL
½ tsp	salt	2 mL

1. In a large saucepan, over medium-high heat, combine garlic, onion, celery, tomatoes with juice, tomato paste, vinegar, sugar, pickling spice, celery seed and salt; cover and bring to a boil. Reduce heat to medium-low and simmer, stirring occasionally, until reduced by half, about 45 minutes. Let cool for 10 minutes.

2. In blender, in batches, blend tomato mixture on high speed until smooth.

3. Press mixture through a fine, stainless steel or non-metallic strainer into clean saucepan; cover and bring to a boil. Reduce heat to medium-low and simmer for 10 minutes.

4. Ladle into hot, sterilized canning jars and seal according to the lid manufacturer's instructions. Store at room temperature for up to 1 year. Or ladle into sterilized jars and store in the refrigerator for up to 1 month.

Tomatillos Ketchup

Tomatillos are small, green fruits that look like tomatoes but are actually a member of the gooseberry family. Green tomatoes, such as green zebra tomatoes, are varieties of (not just unripe) tomatoes. Together they make a slightly sour and spicy green ketchup that is a tasty novelty for hot dogs, grilled chicken or fish.

2 lbs	green tomatoes, peeled and seeded (see tip, page 63)	1 kg
1	can (26 oz/737g) tomatillos, drained	1
3	jalapeño peppers, seeded and coarsely chopped	3
3	cloves garlic, smashed	3
1	green bell pepper, seeded and coarsely chopped	1
1	Cubanelle pepper, seeded and coarsely chopped	1
1	small onion, coarsely chopped	1
⅓ cup	cider vinegar	75 mL
1 tbsp	dried oregano	15 mL
1 tbsp	granulated sugar	15 mL
1 tsp	salt	5 mL

1. Coarsely chop tomatoes and place in Dutch oven over medium-high heat. Add tomatillos, mashing just to crush, jalapeños, garlic, green pepper, Cubanelle pepper, onion, vinegar, oregano, sugar and salt; cover and bring to a boil. Reduce heat to medium-low and simmer, stirring occasionally, until reduced by half, about 45 minutes. Let cool for 10 minutes.

2. In blender, in batches, blend tomato mixture on high speed until smooth.

3. Press mixture through a fine, non-reactive strainer into clean saucepan; cover and bring to a boil. Reduce heat to medium-low and simmer until very thick, about 20 minutes.

4. Ladle into hot, sterilized canning jars and seal according to the lid manufacturer's instructions. Store at room temperature for up to 1 year. Or ladle into sterilized jars and store in the refrigerator for up to 1 month.

*Roasting mushrooms
dries up the extra
liquid and enhances
their slightly smoky,
woodsy taste. This is a
thick, flavorful topping
for a real beef burger
or sausage on a bun.*

Mushroom Ketchup

- *Preheat oven to 400°F (200°C)*
- *13- by 9-inch (3 L) baking pan or dish*

2 lbs	cremini and/or field mushrooms	1 kg
1 tbsp	olive oil	15 mL
½ tsp	salt	2 mL
1 cup	boiling water	250 mL
1 cup	chopped red onion	250 mL
1 cup	white wine vinegar or cider vinegar	250 mL
½ tsp	freshly ground black pepper	2 mL
½ tsp	ground ginger	2 mL
½ tsp	ground allspice	2 mL

1. Wipe mushrooms clean with a damp cloth and place in baking pan. Toss with oil and salt. Roast in preheated oven for 1 hour, or until mushrooms are shriveled and dry and all liquid is evaporated.

2. Scrape mushrooms into a large saucepan. Pour boiling water into baking pan, washing out dried mushroom juices and scraping up any bits; pour into saucepan with mushrooms. Add onion, vinegar, pepper, ginger and allspice; cover and bring to a boil over medium-high heat. Reduce heat to medium-low and simmer, stirring occasionally, for 30 minutes, or until most of the liquid has evaporated.

3. In blender, in batches, blend mushroom mixture on low speed, scraping down sides as necessary, until semi-smooth with no large chunks remaining.

4. Return to saucepan and cook for 10 minutes, until very thick and fragrant. Adjust seasoning, if desired.

5. Ladle into hot, sterilized canning jars and seal according to the lid manufacturer's instructions. Store at room temperature for up to 1 year. Or ladle into sterilized jars and store in the refrigerator for up to 1 month.

Ketchups are not always tomato-based sauces. This sweet-sour concoction tastes like plum sauce and is particularly good with chicken fingers and pork.

Rhubarb Ketchup

2	onions, chopped	2
4 cups	chopped fresh or frozen, thawed rhubarb (about 1 lb/500 g)	1 L
1 cup	packed brown sugar	250 mL
1 cup	granulated sugar	250 mL
1 cup	cider vinegar	250 mL
¼ cup	orange juice	50 mL
2 tsp	salt	10 mL
2 tsp	pickling spice	10 mL
1 tsp	ground cinnamon	5 mL
1 tsp	ground ginger	5 mL
½ tsp	ground allspice (optional)	2 mL

1. In a large saucepan, over medium-high heat, combine onions, rhubarb, brown sugar, granulated sugar, vinegar, orange juice, salt, pickling spice, cinnamon, ginger and allspice, if using; cover and bring to boil. Reduce heat to medium-low and simmer, stirring occasionally, until thick and pulpy, about 45 minutes. Let cool for 10 minutes.

2. In blender, in batches, blend rhubarb mixture on high speed until smooth.

3. Press mixture through a fine, non-reactive strainer into clean saucepan; cover and bring to a boil. Reduce heat to medium-low and simmer until thick, about 10 minutes.

4. Ladle into hot, sterilized canning jars and seal according to the lid manufacturer's instructions. Store for up to 1 year.

Variation

Rhubarb Barbecue Sauce: In a medium saucepan, combine 1 cup (250 mL) Rhubarb Ketchup, 1 cup (250 mL) water, 2 tbsp (25 mL) cider vinegar, 1 tbsp (15 mL) brown sugar, 1 tbsp (15 mL) Worcestershire sauce, ¾ tsp (4 mL) salt, ½ tsp (2 mL) celery seed and a pinch of hot pepper flakes; cover and bring to a boil. Reduce heat and simmer, stirring occasionally, for 25 minutes, or until reduced by half. Store in the refrigerator for up to 1 month. Makes about 1 cup (250 mL).

A sophisticated mustard, especially good for turkey and chicken sandwiches or ground turkey or fish burgers.

White Wine–Tarragon Mustard

¾ cup	white wine	175 mL
½ cup	mustard seeds	125 mL
½ cup	white wine vinegar or tarragon-flavored vinegar	125 mL
1 tbsp	dry mustard	15 mL
2 tsp	crumbled dried tarragon	10 mL
1 tsp	salt	5 mL
1 tsp	granulated sugar	5 mL

1. In a small bowl, stir together wine and mustard seeds. Cover and let stand overnight.

2. In blender, on low speed, blend mustard seeds, vinegar, mustard, tarragon, salt and sugar until creamy, with some seeds remaining, or until desired smoothness.

3. Pour into airtight jars and refrigerate for 4 days before serving. Store in the refrigerator for up to 3 months.

Mustard fumes are very strong, so open the top and let fumes dissipate before peeking inside.

Hot Honey Mustard

1 cup	dry mustard	250 mL
½ cup	liquid honey	125 mL
½ cup	rice or cider vinegar	125 mL
¼ cup	warm water	50 mL
1 tsp	dried thyme	5 mL
½ tsp	salt	2 mL

1. In blender, on high speed, blend mustard, honey, vinegar, water, thyme and salt, scraping down sides as necessary, until smooth.

2. Pour into airtight jars and let stand at room temperature for 3 days before serving. Store in the refrigerator for up to 3 months.

Seed-Style Horseradish Mustard

½ cup	dry mustard	125 mL
¼ cup	mustard seeds	50 mL
½ cup	cider vinegar	125 mL
¼ cup	warm water	50 mL
2 tbsp	drained prepared horseradish	25 mL
1 tsp	salt	5 mL

1. In blender, on low speed, blend mustard, mustard seeds, vinegar, water, horseradish and salt, scraping down sides as necessary, until smooth, with some seeds remaining.

2. Pour into an airtight jar and let stand at room temperature for 3 days before serving. Store in the refrigerator for up to 3 months.

*A thin, sweet mustard
that is deliciously
suited to shaved ham,
smoked turkey or
chicken on very
fresh bread.*

Russian-Style Mustard

1 cup	dry mustard	250 mL
¾ cup	granulated sugar	175 mL
¼ cup	boiling water	50 mL
3 tbsp	white vinegar or white wine vinegar	45 mL
2 tbsp	vegetable oil	25 mL
½ tsp	salt	2 mL

1. In blender, on high speed, blend mustard, sugar, boiling water, vinegar, oil and salt, scraping down sides as necessary, until smooth.

2. Pour into airtight jars and let stand at room temperature for 3 days before serving. Store in the refrigerator for up to 3 months.

Mayonnaise

Nothing compares to homemade mayonnaise. And with a blender, making mayonnaise isn't a daunting task; just remember to have all the ingredients at room temperature.

This recipe contains a raw egg. If the food safety of raw eggs is a concern for you, use the pasteurized liquid whole egg instead.

TIP

If the mayonnaise separates, start again with another egg or ¼ cup (50 mL) pasteurized liquid whole egg, add oil (about 3 tbsp/45 mL) drop by drop until the mixture emulsifies properly, then add the separated mayonnaise in a slow stream.

1	egg, at room temperature (or ¼ cup/50 mL pasteurized liquid whole egg)	1
2 tsp	Dijon mustard	10 mL
2 tsp	white wine vinegar or cider vinegar	10 mL
½ tsp	salt	2 mL
¼ tsp	freshly ground white pepper	1 mL
½ cup	vegetable oil, divided	125 mL
½ cup	extra-virgin olive oil	125 mL
1 tbsp	freshly squeezed lemon juice	15 mL

1. In blender, on low speed, blend egg, mustard, vinegar, salt and pepper.

2. With motor running on high speed, through hole in top, add 3 tbsp (45 mL) of the vegetable oil, one drop at a time. Add remaining vegetable oil and olive oil in a slow stream until thickened, scraping down sides as necessary and pulsing to incorporate oil as mixture thickens. On low speed, pulse in lemon juice.

3. *Make ahead:* Cover and refrigerate for up to 1 week.

Variation

Lemon Pepper Mayonnaise: Prepare mayonnaise as directed above. In a bowl, stir together mayonnaise, ¼ tsp (1 mL) lemon zest, 2 tbsp (25 mL) lemon juice and 2 tsp (10 mL) pepper.

Fines Herbes Mayonnaise

1	clove garlic, chopped	1
1 cup	mayonnaise (store-bought or see recipe, page 54)	250 mL
¼ cup	chopped fresh chives	50 mL
¼ cup	loosely packed parsley leaves	50 mL
2 tbsp	fresh chervil (optional)	25 mL
1 tbsp	chopped shallot	15 mL
2 tsp	fresh tarragon	10 mL
¼ tsp	hot pepper sauce	1 mL

1. In blender, pulse garlic, mayonnaise, chives, parsley, chervil (if using), shallot, tarragon and hot pepper sauce until finely minced.

2. *Make ahead:* Cover and refrigerate for up to 1 week.

This sweet, creamy mayonnaise is excellent as a base for egg or salmon salad or as a topping for poached fish.

This recipe contains a raw egg. If the food safety of raw eggs is a concern for you, use the pasteurized liquid whole egg instead.

Russian-Style Mayonnaise

3	egg yolks (or ⅓ cup/75 mL pasteurized liquid whole egg)	3
2 tbsp	Russian-style mustard	25 mL
1 tbsp	freshly squeezed lemon juice	15 mL
1 tbsp	sour cream	15 mL
½ tsp	granulated sugar	2 mL
½ tsp	salt	2 mL
1 cup	vegetable oil	250 mL
¼ cup	chopped drained capers	50 mL

1. In blender, on low speed, combine egg yolks, mustard, lemon juice, sour cream, sugar and salt. With motor running on high speed, through hole in top, slowly drizzle in oil until thick and smooth, scraping down sides as necessary. Pulse in capers.

2. *Make ahead:* Cover and refrigerate for up to 1 week.

For a fruity sweet-and-sour mayonnaise, increase lime juice to 2 tbsp (25 mL), omit honey and add 2 tbsp (25 mL) mango chutney.

Curry Mayonnaise

1	clove garlic, smashed	1
1 cup	mayonnaise (store-bought or see recipe, page 54)	250 mL
1 tbsp	freshly squeezed lemon juice	15 mL
1 tsp	liquid honey	5 mL
1 tsp	curry paste or curry powder	5 mL
¼ tsp	ground ginger	1 mL
Pinch	ground cumin	Pinch
Pinch	ground cloves	Pinch
Pinch	freshly ground black pepper	Pinch

1. In blender, on low speed, blend garlic, mayonnaise, lemon juice, honey, curry paste, ginger, cumin, cloves and pepper until garlic is minced.

2. *Make ahead:* Cover and refrigerate for up to 1 week.

For a unique, smoky flavor, replace the optional paprika with smoked Spanish paprika.

You can also use 2 tsp (10 mL) fresh tarragon.

Instead of the lemon juice, try 2 tsp (10 mL) cider vinegar.

Tartar Sauce

1 cup	mayonnaise (store-bought or see recipe, page 54)	250 mL
1 tbsp	chopped shallots or red onion	15 mL
1 tbsp	chopped fresh parsley	15 mL
1 tbsp	chopped sweet pickle	15 mL
1 tbsp	chopped dill pickle	15 mL
1 tbsp	chopped drained capers	15 mL
1 tbsp	freshly squeezed lemon juice	15 mL
¾ tsp	dried tarragon	4 mL
1 tsp	Dijon mustard	5 mL
¼ tsp	freshly ground black pepper	1 mL
¼ tsp	sweet paprika (optional)	1 mL
Pinch	cayenne pepper	Pinch

1. In blender, on low speed, blend mayonnaise, shallots, parsley, sweet and dill pickles, capers, lemon juice, tarragon, mustard, pepper, paprika (if using) and cayenne until very finely chopped.

2. *Make ahead:* Cover and refrigerate for up to 1 week.

Sauce Gribiche

2	hard-cooked eggs, quartered	2
⅓ cup	white wine vinegar or cider vinegar	75 mL
1 tsp	Dijon mustard	5 mL
¼ tsp	salt	1 mL
¼ tsp	freshly ground black pepper	1 mL
Dash	hot pepper sauce	Dash
1 cup	extra-virgin olive oil	250 mL
1 tbsp	drained and rinsed capers	15 mL
1 tbsp	chopped fresh parsley	15 mL
2 tsp	chopped chives	10 mL
1 tsp	fresh tarragon (or ¼ tsp/1 mL dried)	5 mL

1. In blender, on low speed, combine eggs, vinegar, mustard, salt, pepper and hot pepper sauce until smooth.

2. With motor running on high speed, though hole in top, pour in oil in a thin stream until incorporated.

3. On low speed, add capers, parsley, chives and tarragon; blend until finely chopped.

4. *Make ahead:* Cover and refrigerate for up to 1 week.

Fresh Basil Oil

1 cup	packed fresh basil leaves	250 mL
2 cups	extra-virgin olive oil	500 mL

1. In blender, on high speed, purée basil and oil.

2. Strain through a coffee filter or cheesecloth into an airtight container and store in the refrigerator for up to 1 week.

*Fresh homemade
hollandaise sauce on
blanched asparagus
is heaven on a plate.
Topping simple
steamed broccoli
or cauliflower, this
egg-rich sauce turns
a pedestrian vegetable
into a luxurious
experience. A blender
makes it as easy as
opening a jar.*

*This recipe contains
raw egg yolks. If the
food safety of raw
eggs is a concern
for you, use the
pasteurized liquid
whole egg instead.*

TIP

Hollandaise sauce is
essential for Eggs
Benedict: Place 1 slice
of ham or back bacon
on a toasted English
muffin half, top
with poached
egg and smother in
hollandaise sauce.

Hollandaise Sauce

½ cup	unsalted butter	125 mL
3	egg yolks (or ⅓ cup/75 mL pasteurized liquid whole egg)	3
2 tbsp	freshly squeezed lemon juice	25 mL
¼ tsp	salt	1 mL
Pinch	cayenne pepper	Pinch
Pinch	freshly ground white pepper	Pinch

1. In a small saucepan, heat butter until bubbling but not browned.

2. In blender, on high speed, blend egg yolks, lemon juice, salt, cayenne and white pepper until smooth, about 5 seconds. With motor running, through hole in top, pour in butter in a thin stream until incorporated, about 30 seconds. Continue blending until smooth, about 5 seconds.

3. To keep warm, place in a heatproof bowl over hot, not boiling, water.

Use aioli for fish, boiled meats, boiled potatoes or beets, or as a dip for vegetable crudités. For an even more garlicky aioli, add up to 4 more garlic cloves, but beware of the bite!

This recipe contains raw eggs. If the food safety of raw eggs is a concern for you, replace the whole egg and the egg yolk with ⅓ cup (75 mL) pasteurized liquid whole egg.

TIPS

All ingredients should be at room temperature.

Substitute 1 anchovy fillet, rinsed and drained, for the salt.

Aioli

1	slice white bread, crusts removed and cubed	1
	Water, for soaking	
4	cloves garlic, smashed	4
1	whole egg	1
1	egg yolk	1
¼ tsp	salt	1 mL
Pinch	freshly ground black pepper	Pinch
1 cup	extra-virgin olive oil	250 mL
2 tsp	freshly squeezed lemon juice	10 mL
1 tbsp	cold water (approx.)	15 mL

1. In a shallow bowl, sprinkle bread with water until soaked, then squeeze dry.

2. In blender, on low speed, blend bread, garlic, egg, egg yolk, salt and pepper, scraping down sides as necessary, until smooth.

3. With motor running on high speed, through hole in top, pour in oil in a very thin stream until incorporated and sauce is thick.

4. On low speed, add lemon juice. Thin with cold water as necessary for desired consistency.

5. *Make ahead:* Cover and refrigerate for up to 1 week.

Pesto

Ever since North Americans discovered this Genoese sauce about 30 years ago, its popularity has never abated.

TIPS

To toast nuts, fry in a small skillet over medium heat, tossing often, until lightly colored, about 4 minutes.

Pesto can be frozen after Step 1 for up to 6 months in an airtight container.

Toss with fresh-cooked pasta (add 2 tbsp/25 mL softened butter and 1 to 2 tbsp/15 to 25 mL hot pasta water) or use as a versatile flavoring base. Makes enough for 1½ lbs (750 g) pasta, or 6 servings.

2	cloves garlic, smashed	2
2 cups	loosely packed torn fresh basil leaves	500 mL
½ cup	extra-virgin olive oil	125 mL
2 tbsp	lightly toasted pine nuts	25 mL
1 tsp	salt	5 mL
⅔ cup	freshly grated Parmesan cheese (or ⅓ cup/75 mL each Parmesan and pecorino cheese)	150 mL

1. In blender, on high speed, purée garlic, basil, oil, pine nuts and salt, scraping down sides as necessary. Pulse in cheese.

2. *Make ahead:* Cover and refrigerate for up to 3 days.

I love the flavor of peppery arugula with salty and piquant pecorino cheese.

TIP

Add to 4 servings of hot pasta with a little pasta cooking water to thin and 2 tbsp (25 mL) butter, if desired. If you wish, you can replace the butter with the same amount of yogurt or cream.

Arugula and Walnut Pesto

1	clove garlic, smashed	1
2 cups	loosely packed arugula	500 mL
½ cup	lightly toasted walnuts (see tip, page 60)	125 mL
⅓ cup	extra-virgin olive oil	75 mL
½ cup	pecorino or other hard sheep's milk cheese	125 mL

1. In blender, on low speed, blend garlic, arugula and walnuts, scraping down sides as necessary, until finely chopped. With motor running, through hole in top, pour in oil in a thin stream until incorporated and pesto is a fine consistency. Pulse in pecorino cheese.

2. *Make ahead:* Cover and refrigerate for up to 3 days.

This garlicky Mediterranean sauce is wonderful on boiled potatoes, pasta salads or grilled fish.

Anchovy Pistou

6	anchovy fillets	6
5	cloves garlic, smashed	5
½ cup	loosely packed basil leaves	125 mL
¼ cup	loosely packed parsley leaves	50 mL
¼ cup	extra-virgin olive oil	50 mL
¼ tsp	freshly ground black pepper	1 mL

1. In blender, on low speed, blend anchovies, garlic, basil, parsley, oil and pepper until very finely chopped.

2. *Make ahead:* Cover and refrigerate for up to 3 days.

This nutty puréed sauce is similar to pesto and can be used in the same way. It is particularly nice on grilled meats and fish.

Pumpkin Seed Herb Sauce

⅓ cup	raw shelled pumpkin seeds	75 mL
1	small red or green hot pepper	1
1	clove garlic, minced	1
1 cup	lightly packed fresh cilantro	250 mL
½ cup	lightly packed fresh parsley	125 mL
3 tbsp	freshly squeezed lime juice	45 mL
3 tbsp	pumpkin seed oil or extra-virgin olive oil	45 mL
2 tbsp	water	25 mL
¼ tsp	salt	1 mL

1. In a skillet, over medium heat, toast pumpkin seeds, shaking pan often, until popping starts to subside and seeds are golden, about 5 minutes.

2. In blender, on high speed, purée toasted pumpkin seeds, hot pepper, garlic, cilantro, parsley, lime juice, oil, water and salt, scraping down sides as necessary.

3. *Make ahead:* Cover and refrigerate for up to 3 days.

When you have wonderfully ripe and tasty red or black tomatoes (such as black Krims or black Germans), make this simple sauce to toss with hot pasta. Add some chopped bocconcini cheese and freshly grated Parmesan, if desired.

Uncooked Fresh Tomato Sauce

1 lb	very ripe tomatoes, peeled and seeded (see tip, page 63)	500 g
¼ cup	loosely packed fresh basil leaves (or ½ tsp/2 mL dried oregano)	50 mL
3 tbsp	extra-virgin olive oil	45 mL
½ tsp	salt	2 mL
Pinch	freshly ground black pepper	Pinch

1. In blender, on low speed, blend tomatoes, basil, oil, salt and pepper until slightly chunky.

Make sauce in late summer. To keep it over the winter, freeze it or preserve it (see tip, below).

TIPS

Recipe can be doubled or tripled.

To preserve: Transfer sauce to a 4-cup (1 L) canning jar. Stir in $\frac{1}{2}$ tsp (2 mL) citric acid and seal with a 2-piece lid. Process in a boiling water bath for 20 minutes. Make sure lid is sealed and store in a cool place for up to 1 year. Use up within 3 days of opening.

To peel and seed tomatoes, blanch in boiling water until skins begin to peel away, about 15 seconds. With a slotted spoon, remove tomatoes and place in ice water. With a paring knife, peel off skin, then scrape out seeds with a spoon.

Fresh Tomato Sauce

3 lbs	very ripe tomatoes, peeled (see tip, at left)	1.5 kg
$\frac{1}{4}$ cup	extra-virgin olive oil	50 mL
3	cloves garlic, minced	3
1 tsp	salt	5 mL
$\frac{1}{4}$ tsp	freshly ground black pepper	1 mL
1	bay leaf (optional)	1

1. Into a sieve over a bowl, squeeze out seeds from tomatoes; drain juice into bowl and discard seeds.

2. Transfer tomatoes and juice to blender in batches and purée on high speed.

3. In a large saucepan, heat oil over medium heat. Add garlic, salt and pepper; cook, stirring, for 1 to 2 minutes, until garlic is fragrant but not colored. Add tomatoes and bay leaf, if using; reduce heat and simmer, uncovered, stirring occasionally, until mixture is cooked down to about 4 cups (1 L), about 20 minutes. Remove bay leaf.

4. Make ahead: Transfer sauce to freezer bags or airtight containers and freeze for up to 6 months or preserve (see tip, at left).

5. To serve, reheat in a pot over medium heat until hot and bubbling.

Variations

Fresh Tomato Marinara Sauce: With garlic, add 1 finely chopped small onion, 3 chopped anchovy fillets and $\frac{1}{4}$ tsp (1 mL) hot pepper flakes. With tomatoes, add 1 tsp (5 mL) dried oregano.

Fresh Tomato Sauce with Basil: To blender, add $\frac{1}{4}$ cup (50 mL) loosely packed fresh basil. Before serving, add 2 to 3 torn fresh basil leaves per serving and cook for 30 seconds.

Fresh Tomato Sauce with Fennel Seed: To either Fresh Tomato Marinara Sauce, or Fresh Tomato Sauce with Basil, add 1 tsp (5 mL) lightly crushed fennel seeds to oil 30 seconds before adding garlic.

**MAKES ABOUT
2 CUPS (500 ML)**

*Roasting tomatoes
gives them a very
intense and sweet
flavor. Use ripe
tomatoes — red,
yellow or orange.*

Roasted Tomato Sauce

● *Preheat oven to 400°F (200°C)*
● *Baking dish*

2 lbs	very ripe tomatoes	1 kg
2	cloves garlic, minced	2
1 tsp	salt	5 mL
¼ tsp	freshly ground black pepper	1 mL
Pinch	granulated sugar	Pinch
⅓ cup	extra-virgin olive oil	75 mL

1. Slice tomatoes in half and place them cut side up in a baking dish just big enough to hold them. Sprinkle garlic over tomatoes, and press it down into them. Sprinkle with salt and pepper and sugar, then drizzle with oil. Bake in preheated oven for 1½ to 2 hours, or until soft and shriveled but not dried out.

2. Transfer to blender and purée on high speed.

3. *Make ahead:* Cover and refrigerate for up to 3 days.

**MAKES ABOUT
1½ CUPS (375 ML)**

*Spread pizza dough
with this sauce. Top
with grated pecorino
cheese, such as Romano,
or fresh mozzarella,
and anchovy filets,
if desired.*

Fresh Fennel Tomato Pizza Sauce

1	bulb fennel	1
2	tomatoes, chopped	2
2	cloves garlic, chopped	2
¼ cup	loosely packed basil leaves (or ½ tsp/2 mL dried oregano)	50 mL
¼ cup	extra-virgin olive oil	50 mL
½ tsp	salt	2 mL
¼ tsp	freshly ground black pepper	1 mL

1. Trim stalks and fronds from fennel. Quarter fennel bulb and blanch in a large pot of boiling salted water until tender, about 8 minutes; drain.

2. In blender, on high speed, purée fennel, tomatoes, garlic, basil, oil, salt and pepper until smooth.

3. *Make ahead:* Cover and refrigerate for up to 3 days.

Spanish Tomato Sauce

**MAKES ABOUT
2 CUPS (500 ML)**

*The combination of
fragrant Spanish
paprika with ripe
tomatoes is irresistible.
Try it with shrimp
(sauté shrimp quickly
in a little olive oil, then
finish cooking with
some tomato sauce and
chopped fresh parsley)
or in other dishes that
call for tomato sauce.*

TIP

If ripe tomatoes
aren't available, use
a 28-oz (796 g) can
of peeled tomatoes.

2 tbsp	extra-virgin olive oil	25 mL
2	cloves garlic, minced	2
1	onion, chopped	1
1	bay leaf	1
1 ½ tsp	smoked or sweet Spanish paprika	7 mL
1 tsp	sherry vinegar	5 mL
1 ½ lbs	very ripe tomatoes, chopped	750 g
¾ tsp	salt	4 mL
Pinch	granulated sugar	Pinch

1. In a large saucepan, heat oil over medium heat. Add garlic and onion; cook, stirring occasionally, until onion is translucent and soft, about 5 minutes. Stir in bay leaf and paprika. Add vinegar and give mixture a good stir, then add tomatoes, salt and sugar. Simmer for 20 minutes, until thickened. Remove bay leaf.

2. Transfer to blender and blend on low speed until smooth. Push through a sieve to remove seeds and peel.

3. *Make ahead:* Cover and refrigerate for up to 3 days.

Tomato-Pepper Sauce

**MAKES ABOUT
1½ CUPS (375 ML)**

*Drizzle this fresh
gazpacho-flavored
sauce over hot poached
or grilled fish or
chicken. Or serve over
cold chicken, veal or
fish on a bed of greens
for a light summer
lunch or supper, or
as a first course.*

3	tomatoes, peeled and seeded	3
½	white or sweet onion, chopped	½
1	green bell pepper, chopped	1
1	stalk celery, chopped	1
¼ cup	loosely packed fresh parsley	50 mL
2 tbsp	extra-virgin olive oil	25 mL
1 tbsp	red wine vinegar	15 mL
½ tsp	salt	2 mL
¼ tsp	freshly ground black pepper	1 mL
Dash	hot pepper sauce	Dash

1. In blender, on low speed, blend tomatoes, onion, bell pepper, celery, parsley, oil, vinegar, salt, pepper and hot pepper sauce until almost smooth.

2. *Make ahead:* Cover and refrigerate for up to 3 days.

TIP

Seed all or half of the dried red hot peppers for a milder sauce.

Indonesian Spicy Tomato Sauce

$\frac{1}{4}$ cup	broken dried red hot peppers	50 mL
$\frac{1}{3}$ cup	warm water	75 mL
2	cloves garlic, chopped	2
1 cup	diced seeded drained canned tomatoes	250 mL
$1\frac{1}{2}$ tsp	granulated sugar	7 mL
$1\frac{1}{2}$ tsp	rice vinegar	7 mL
1 tsp	salt	5 mL
2 tbsp	peanut oil	25 mL
3	whole cloves	3
$\frac{1}{2}$ tsp	fennel seeds	2 mL
$\frac{1}{4}$ tsp	ground cumin	1 mL

1. In blender, soak hot peppers in warm water until soft, about 1 hour. Add garlic, tomatoes, sugar, vinegar and salt; blend until smooth.

2. In a skillet, heat oil over medium heat. Add cloves, fennel seeds and cumin; cook, shaking pan, until seeds begin to pop, about 30 seconds. Add hot pepper mixture. Reduce heat to low and cook, stirring often, until about half the liquid is evaporated and mixture is a thick ketchup-like sauce, about 15 minutes. Let cool.

3. Store in the refrigerator for up to 2 weeks.

*Serve this tasty sauce
over grilled steak or
roast beef. It is also
an excellent sauce for
lamb or pork chops.*

Mushroom Sauce for Beef

2 tbsp	butter or extra-virgin olive oil	25 mL
3	anchovies, chopped	3
1	small onion, chopped	1
1	clove garlic, minced	1
2 cups	halved mushrooms (about 6 oz/175 g)	500 mL
¾ tsp	chopped fresh thyme (or ¼ tsp/1 mL dried)	4 mL
2 tbsp	all-purpose flour	25 mL
½ cup	dry red wine	125 mL
½ cup	beef stock	125 mL
¼ tsp	salt	1 mL
¼ tsp	freshly ground black pepper	1 mL
2 tbsp	minced fresh parsley	25 mL

1. In a medium saucepan, melt butter (or heat oil) over medium-high heat. Add anchovies, onion and garlic; cook, stirring, for 4 to 5 minutes, or until onion is golden. Reduce heat to medium and add mushrooms and thyme. Cook, stirring often, for 4 to 5 minutes, or until mushrooms are tender and lightly browned. Stir in flour and cook, stirring, until flour no longer smells raw, about 1 minute.

2. Scrape into blender and add wine, stock, salt and pepper. Blend on low speed, scraping down sides as necessary, until mushrooms are finely chopped.

3. Return to saucepan. Bring to a simmer over medium-low heat and simmer for 4 to 5 minutes, or until very thick. Stir in parsley.

4. *Make ahead:* Cover and refrigerate for up to 3 days.

*Serve this rich sauce
with poached or roasted
chicken. It is also
suitable for veal chops
or pork tenderloin.*

Mushroom Sauce for Poultry

2 tbsp	butter	25 mL
1	small onion, chopped	1
1	clove garlic, minced	1
2 cups	halved mushrooms (about 6 oz/175 g)	500 mL
1 tsp	minced fresh tarragon (or 1/2 tsp/2 mL dried)	5 mL
2 tbsp	all-purpose flour	25 mL
1/2 cup	dry white vermouth or dry white wine	125 mL
1/2 cup	chicken stock	125 mL
1/2 tsp	salt	2 mL
1/4 tsp	freshly ground white pepper	1 mL
1/4 cup	whipping (35%) cream	50 mL
Pinch	ground nutmeg	Pinch
2 tbsp	minced fresh parsley	25 mL

1. In a medium saucepan, melt butter over medium-high heat. Add onion and garlic; cook, stirring, for 4 to 5 minutes, or until onion is golden. Reduce heat to medium and add mushrooms and tarragon. Cook, stirring often, for 4 to 5 minutes, or until mushrooms are tender and lightly browned. Stir in flour and cook, stirring, until flour no longer smells raw, about 1 minute.

2. Scrape into blender and add vermouth, stock, salt and pepper. Blend on low speed, scraping down sides as necessary, until mushrooms are finely chopped.

3. Return to saucepan. Bring to a simmer over medium-low heat and simmer for 4 to 5 minutes, or until very thick. Add whipping cream and nutmeg; simmer for 2 minutes. Stir in parsley.

4. *Make ahead:* Cover and refrigerate for up to 3 days.

This is a lovely sauce for cold poached salmon or chicken, especially on a bed of Belgian endive or watercress.

Cucumber Sauce

¾ cup	sour cream	175 mL
¼ tsp	salt	1 mL
¼ tsp	sweet paprika	1 mL
Pinch	granulated sugar	Pinch
Dash	hot pepper sauce	Dash
3 tbsp	extra-virgin olive oil	45 mL
2 tbsp	sherry vinegar	25 mL
1¼ cup	chopped, seeded and peeled cucumber	300 mL
¼ cup	chopped red onion	50 mL
1 tbsp	minced fresh dill or parsley	15 mL

1. In blender, on high speed, whip sour cream, salt, paprika, sugar and hot pepper sauce until thick. With motor running, through hole in top, pour in oil in a thin stream until incorporated, then pour in vinegar and blend until smooth. Add cucumber and onion; blend on low speed until very finely chopped. Pulse in dill.

2. *Make ahead:* Cover and refrigerate for up to 3 days.

This Greek and Middle Eastern sauce is served simply with bread or warm pitas, as a sauce for grilled meats and as a general garnish at the table. You can use low-fat yogurt if desired, but full-fat Balkan-style yogurt gives the best results.

Cucumber Yogurt Sauce

2	cloves garlic, smashed	2
1	field cucumber, peeled, seeded and chopped	1
2 cups	plain yogurt	500 mL
1 tbsp	freshly squeezed lemon juice	15 mL
¼ cup	loosely packed mint leaves (or 1 tsp/5 mL dried mint)	50 mL
½ tsp	salt	2 mL
	Extra-virgin olive oil	
¼ tsp	cayenne pepper or paprika	1 mL

1. In blender, on low speed, blend garlic, cucumber, yogurt, lemon juice, mint and salt until finely chopped. Scrape into a bowl, drizzle with oil and sprinkle with cayenne.

2. *Make ahead:* Cover and refrigerate for up to 3 days.

Drizzle this Indonesian sauce over a salad of sliced vegetables, such as carrots, cucumber, blanched celery, bean sprouts and green beans, or over sliced fruit, such as pineapple, star fruit (carambola) or pears.

TIP

Dried shrimp are available at Chinese, Southeast Asian and Latin grocers.

Tart Peanut Sauce

¼ cup	dried shrimp	50 mL
⅓ cup	natural crunchy peanut butter	75 mL
¼ cup	freshly squeezed lime juice	50 mL
¼ cup	rice or cider vinegar	50 mL
1 tbsp	chopped Thai bird chilies	15 mL
1 tbsp	soy sauce	15 mL
2 tbsp	granulated sugar	25 mL
2 tbsp	water	25 mL
¼ tsp	salt	1 mL
¼ tsp	freshly ground white pepper	1 mL

1. Soak dried shrimp in cold water for 30 minutes. Drain. In a dry skillet, over medium heat, cook shrimp for 4 to 5 minutes, or until well toasted.

2. Transfer to blender and add peanut butter, lime juice, vinegar, chilies, soy sauce, sugar, water, salt and pepper; purée on high speed.

3. *Make ahead:* Cover and refrigerate for up to 1 week.

A great Thai all-purpose, but very hot, chili sauce.

Chili Vinegar Sauce

1 cup	rice vinegar	250 mL
3 tbsp	fish sauce	45 mL
3 tbsp	water	45 mL
4 tsp	granulated sugar	20 mL
½ tsp	salt	2 mL
5	cloves garlic, chopped	5
8 oz	mixed Thai red and green chilies	250 g
2 tbsp	chopped fresh cilantro	25 mL
1 tbsp	chopped gingerroot	15 mL

1. In a small saucepan, over high heat, bring vinegar, fish sauce, water, sugar and salt to a boil; cook until sugar is dissolved. Let cool slightly.

2. Transfer to blender and add garlic, Thai chilies, cilantro and ginger. Blend on low speed until finely chopped.

3. Store in the refrigerator for up to 1 month.

There are as many variations of hot sauce made with the wickedly hot Scotch bonnet or habanero peppers as there are cooks in the Caribbean. This is a really good one, based on a sauce made by a friend originally from Trinidad. Wear rubber gloves when seeding the hot peppers.

TIP

Cane vinegar (made from sugar cane) is available at some West Indian, Chinese, Southeast Asian, Indian and Pakistani grocers and at all Filipino grocers.

Scotch Bonnet Hot Sauce

1 tbsp	vegetable oil	15 mL
½ cup	seeded halved red, green and yellow Scotch bonnet peppers	125 mL
3	cloves garlic, chopped	3
1	small white onion, chopped	1
½ cup	cane or cider vinegar	125 mL
3 tbsp	granulated sugar	45 mL
1 tsp	salt	5 mL
¼ tsp	ground nutmeg	1 mL
¼ tsp	ground cloves	1 mL
¼ cup	yellow or Dijon mustard	50 mL

1. In a skillet, heat oil over medium heat. Add peppers and cook, stirring, until beginning to soften, about 2 minutes. Add garlic and onion; cook, stirring, for 4 to 5 minutes, or until onion is soft. Add vinegar, sugar, salt, nutmeg and cloves; bring to a boil and cook, stirring, until sugar is dissolved. Remove from heat and let cool.

2. Scrape into blender, add mustard and blend on low speed, scraping down sides as necessary, until finely chopped.

3. Scrape into a sterilized glass jar and store in the refrigerator for up to 6 months.

This hot sauce is an ubiquitous condiment for North African dishes. For a milder sauce, seed the chilies before soaking.

Harissa

½ cup	small dried red chilies	125 mL
	Warm water	
2 tbsp	coriander seeds	25 mL
1 tbsp	cumin seeds	15 mL
1 tbsp	caraway seeds	15 mL
¼ cup	freshly squeezed lemon juice	50 mL
1½ tsp	salt	7 mL
½ cup	extra-virgin olive oil	125 mL

1. In a bowl, cover chilies with warm water. Let soak until soft, about 1 hour.

2. Meanwhile, in a skillet, over medium-low heat, toast coriander seeds, shaking pan, until slightly darkened and fragrant, about 3 minutes. Set aside. In same skillet, toast cumin and caraway seeds, shaking pan, for 1 to 2 minutes, or until fragrant and wiggling about in pan.

3. In blender, on high speed, grind toasted coriander, cumin and caraway seeds to a fine powder.

4. Drain chilies and add to blender with lemon juice and salt. Blend on high speed until fairly smooth. With motor running, through hole in top, pour in oil in a thin stream until incorporated.

5. Scrape into a sterilized glass jar and store in the refrigerator for up to 3 months.

This is my favorite chili sauce for roasted and grilled meats and fish. Be warned, it's very hot.

Thai Cooked Chili Sauce

4 oz	green Thai chilies or other green hot peppers	125 g
4 oz	red Thai chilies or other red hot peppers	125 g
1 tbsp	vegetable oil	15 mL
4	cloves garlic, chopped	4
½ cup	chopped red onions	125 mL
1 tbsp	chopped cilantro root (or 4 tsp/20 mL chopped fresh cilantro stems)	15 mL
2 tsp	crushed palm sugar or light brown sugar	10 mL
1 tsp	freshly ground white pepper	5 mL
3 tbsp	freshly squeezed lime juice	45 mL
2 tbsp	fish sauce	25 mL
	Finely chopped fresh cilantro	

1. If using large hot peppers, cut into a few pieces each (leave Thai chilies whole).

2. In a nonstick skillet, heat oil over medium heat. Add chilies, garlic, onions and cilantro; cook, stirring, until vegetables are soft and fragrant, about 7 minutes. Stir in sugar and pepper; cook for 1 minute. Remove from heat and let cool.

3. Transfer to blender and add lime juice and fish sauce. Blend on low speed, scraping down sides as necessary, to a coarse paste.

4. Store in the refrigerator for up to 4 weeks.

5. To serve, mix 3 tbsp (45 mL) of the chili sauce with 1 tsp (5 mL) finely chopped fresh cilantro.

*This hot, smoky sauce
is delicious with
hamburgers, fish or
tortilla chips. Blend
longer for a smooth
sauce; less for
chunky salsa.*

Chipotle Chili Sauce

3	jalapeño peppers, seeded and roughly chopped	3
1½	green bell peppers, seeded and roughly chopped	1½
1	Cubanelle peppers, seeded and roughly chopped	1
1	onion, roughly chopped	1
1	cloves garlic, minced	1
1	can (28 oz/796 mL) diced tomatoes, with juice	1
½	can (6½ oz/200 g) chipotle peppers in adobo sauce	½
½	can (5½ oz/156 mL) tomato paste	½
½ cup	cider vinegar	125 mL
1 tbsp	dried oregano, crumbled	15 mL
1 tbsp	granulated sugar	15 mL
2 tsp	salt	10 mL
¼ cup	chopped fresh cilantro	50 mL

1. In a large saucepan, over medium-high heat, combine jalapeños, green peppers, Cubanelle peppers, onion, garlic, tomatoes with juice, chipotles, tomato paste, vinegar, oregano, sugar and salt; cover and bring to a boil. Reduce heat to medium-low and simmer, stirring occasionally, until thickened and reduced by half, about 45 minutes. Let cool for 10 minutes.

2. In blender, in batches, pulse tomato mixture until semi-smooth, with no large chunks remaining.

3. Return sauce to a clean saucepan and stir in cilantro. Cover and bring to boil; reduce heat to medium-low and simmer 10 minutes.

4. Ladle into hot, sterilized canning jars, process in a water bath, and seal according to the lid manufacturer's instructions. Store for up to 1 year. Refrigerate after opening and use within 1 month.

This eminently simple sauce is wonderful with fried chicken, fish and pork. For a milder sauce, seed the hot peppers.

Malay Sweet-and-Sour Chili Sauce

2	small cloves garlic, chopped	2
1/3 cup	granulated sugar	75 mL
1/3 cup	rice vinegar	75 mL
3 tbsp	freshly squeezed lemon juice	45 mL
1 1/2 tsp	salt	7 mL
15	finger chilies, chopped	15

1. In blender, on low speed, blend garlic, sugar, vinegar, lemon juice and salt until sugar is dissolved. Add hot peppers and blend until finely chopped.

2. Scrape into a sterilized glass jar and store in the refrigerator for up to 1 week.

This Chilean spicy sauce and marinade, similar to Argentina's chimichurri (see variation, below), is a perfect accompaniment to barbecued meats, especially fresh chorizo sausage.

TIP

To make chimichurri, replace cilantro with parsley.

Pebre

2	green onions, finely chopped	2
2	jalapeño peppers, seeded and chopped	2
1 cup	packed fresh cilantro	250 mL
1 cup	packed fresh parsley	250 mL
1/2 cup	water	125 mL
2	cloves garlic, minced	2
1/4 cup	corn oil or olive oil	50 mL
2 tbsp	sherry vinegar or red wine vinegar	25 mL
2 tbsp	freshly squeezed lime juice	25 mL
1/4 tsp	salt	1 mL
2	tomatoes, finely diced	2

1. In blender, pulse onions, jalapeños, cilantro, parsley and water until finely chopped. Pulse in garlic, oil, vinegar, lime juice and salt until blended.

2. *Make ahead:* Cover and refrigerate for up to 3 days.

3. Before serving, stir in tomatoes.

**MAKES ABOUT
3 CUPS (750 ML)**

*Use this marinade for
pork, chicken, capon
or lamb.*

TIPS

Substitute canned
chipotle peppers in
adobo for the dried
and add with the
spices in Step 2.

Makes enough
marinade for 6 lbs
(3 kg) pork, 3 whole
chickens, 2 capons
or 8 lbs (4 kg) chicken
parts, 2 lamb shoulders
or 1 large leg of lamb.
Coat the meat or
poultry with marinade,
cover and refrigerate
overnight. Bring to
room temperature,
then roast in a 350°F
(180°C) oven. Mix
½ cup (125 mL) of the
remaining marinade
with ¼ cup (50 mL)
minced fresh cilantro
and an extra squeeze
of lime juice to
baste during the
last 30 minutes of
cooking. (Or roast
meat or poultry until
it is almost done,
then finish on the
grill, basting for the
last 15 minutes).

Mexican Red Chili Roasting Marinade

5	mild New Mexico chilies or pasilla chilies, seeded	5
3	dried ancho chilies, seeded	3
2	dried chipotle peppers, seeded	2
2 cups	boiling water	500 mL
2	cloves garlic	2
½	Spanish or sweet onion, chopped	½
2 tbsp	freshly squeezed lime juice	25 mL
2 tsp	dried Mexican, Italian or Greek oregano	10 mL
2 tsp	ground coriander	10 mL
1 tsp	salt	5 mL
1 tsp	ground cumin	5 mL
¾ tsp	ground cinnamon	4 mL
½ tsp	freshly ground black pepper	2 mL

1. Break New Mexico, ancho and chipotle chilies into pieces. Place in blender with boiling water. Cover and let sit for 30 minutes or until softened.

2. Purée chilies and water on high speed. Add garlic, onion, lime juice, oregano, coriander, salt, cumin, cinnamon and pepper; purée on high speed.

3. *Make ahead:* Cover and refrigerate for up to 3 days.

This sauce from southern France can be added to soups to pique the flavor or can be used as a spread for crackers or crudités.

Red Pepper Rouille

¼ cup	boiling water	50 mL
1 to 2	dried hot red peppers, seeded	1 to 2
1	slice white bread, crusts removed	1
3	cloves garlic, smashed	3
1	roasted red bell pepper, peeled	1
¼ tsp	salt	1 mL
¼ cup	extra-virgin olive oil	50 mL

1. Soak dried peppers in boiling water for 15 minutes. Drain, reserving 2 tbsp (25 mL) of the soaking water.

2. Meanwhile, cube bread; in a bowl, sprinkle bread with water until soaked, then squeeze dry.

3. In blender, on low speed, blend hot peppers, bread, garlic, red pepper, soaking water and salt until smooth. With motor running, through hole in top, pour in oil in a thin stream until incorporated.

4. *Make ahead:* Cover and refrigerate for up to 1 week.

Use Saffron Rouille as you would Red Pepper Rouille. All ingredients should be at room temperature.

This recipe contains raw eggs. If the food safety of raw eggs is a concern for you, replace the whole egg and the egg yolk with ⅓ cup (75 mL) pasteurized liquid whole egg.

Saffron Rouille

½ tsp	saffron threads, crumbled	2 mL
1 tbsp	hot water	15 mL
3	cloves garlic, smashed	3
1	whole egg	1
1	egg yolk	1
¼ tsp	cayenne pepper	1 mL
¼ tsp	salt	1 mL
1 cup	extra-virgin olive oil	250 mL
2 tbsp	freshly squeezed lemon juice	25 mL

1. In a small bowl, soak saffron in hot water; let cool.

2. In blender, on low speed, blend garlic, egg, egg yolk, cayenne and salt until smooth. With motor running, through hole in top, pour in oil in a thin stream until incorporated. Blend in saffron mixture and lemon juice.

3. *Make ahead:* Cover and refrigerate for up to 3 days.

This is my favorite curry spice mixture.

TIP

Watch carefully while toasting spices, as they will become bitter if over-toasted. Each of the spices will take a different amount of time to toast properly. Coriander seeds will take about 3 to 4 minutes to toast, while cumin seed will toast very quickly. Spices are ready when they are very fragrant and turn a few shades deeper in color (except for fenugreek, which should be very lightly toasted). Cayenne and turmeric must be constantly stirred while toasting.

Malay Curry Powder

3 tbsp	coriander seeds	45 mL
7 tsp	fennel seeds	35 mL
2 tbsp	ground turmeric	25 mL
1 tbsp	cayenne pepper	15 mL
4 tsp	cumin seeds	20 mL
2 tsp	anise seeds	10 mL
1½ tsp	whole cloves	7 mL
1 tsp	fenugreek seeds	5 mL
1 tsp	white peppercorns	5 mL
½ tsp	black peppercorns	2 mL
3	2-inch (5 cm) pieces Asian cinnamon (cassia bark), broken into small pieces	3
½	whole nutmeg, cut or crushed into smaller bits	½
6	whole green cardamom pods	6
3	black cardamom pods, seeds only (about ½ tsp/2 mL)	3

1. In a dry heavy-bottomed skillet wiped clean of any lingering oil, over medium-low heat, separately toast coriander seeds, fennel seeds, turmeric, cayenne, cumin seeds, anise seeds, cloves, fenugreek seeds, white and black peppercorns, Asian cinnamon and nutmeg, shaking them around a bit for even toasting, until fragrant and slightly darkened (each will take a different time to toast properly; see tip, at left). Remove immediately to a plate to cool.

2. In blender, on high speed, blend toasted spices, green cardamom pods and black cardamom seeds to a fine powder. Push through a fine sieve, then re-blend any coarser bits left in the sieve. Mix together thoroughly and let cool completely.

3. Transfer to a bottle and store for up to 6 months.

Armenian Pepper Paste

*Make this mildly hot
pepper paste in the
autumn when the
local pepper harvest
is available. Use it
as you would tomato
paste in stews,
sauces and soups.
The flavor is incredibly
intense, due to the
concentration from
the cooking method.*

TIP

The citric acid (sour
salt) helps preserve
the fresh flavor
of the paste.

- Preheat oven to 350°F (180°C)
- 13- by 9-inch (3 L) baking dish

5 lbs	red bell peppers	2.5 kg
10	large hot red peppers, such as hot Sheppard peppers	10
	Boiling water	
½ cup	freshly squeezed lemon juice	125 mL
4 tsp	salt	20 mL
Pinch	citric acid	Pinch
¼ cup	olive oil (approx.)	50 mL

1. Seed and remove inner membranes from bell and hot peppers. Place in a large saucepan and cover with ¾ inch (2 cm) boiling water. Boil over high heat for 5 minutes.

2. Transfer to blender in batches and purée on high speed.

3. Scrape into baking dish. Bake in preheated oven, scraping down sides and stirring often, for 2½ to 3 hours, or until the consistency of tomato paste. Let cool. Stir in lemon juice, salt and citric acid.

4. Scrape into sterilized glass jars and cover with thin layer of olive oil, replenishing oil each time the paste is used. Store in the refrigerator for up 3 months.

THE BLENDER HAS taken a lot of the work out of making curry pastes. There's no longer any need to use a mortar and pestle. Unlike a food processor, a blender can crush chili seeds and lemon grass to make real pastes. There are innumerable curry pastes in South and Southeast Asia. On pages 80–82, I have chosen to highlight three basic Thai pastes necessary for a large range of Thai dishes. These recipes make a fairly large amount, but you can freeze the pastes in convenient pre-measured amounts (see tip, page 80) for up to 6 months. Halve the recipes if you want to, but paste is easier to blend as a larger quantity.

Later in the book, you will find recipes for three Indian favorites that include curry pastes: Goan Fish Curry (page 159), Shrimp Balchao (page 164) and Chicken Tikka (page 148).

For the best and freshest-tasting Thai curries, make your own paste. Use this one in any recipe that calls for Thai green curry paste, particularly chicken and vegetable curries.

TIPS

Galangal can be purchased at Asian grocers.

Toast seeds in a dry heavy-bottomed skillet wiped clean of any lingering oil over medium-high heat until slightly darkened and fragrant, 3 to 4 minutes for coriander, 1 to 2 minutes for cumin and fennel seeds.

To freeze: Place tablespoon-size (15 mL) dollops in plastic wrap, twist to wrap, then place in a freezer bag.

Thai Green Curry Paste

20	green Thai chilies	20
6	cloves garlic, smashed	6
2	large sprigs fresh cilantro (including roots), chopped	2
2	finely chopped fresh bay leaves (or 1/2 tsp/2 mL ground dried)	2
2/3 cup	chopped shallots	150 mL
1/4 cup	finely chopped lemon grass (white and light green parts only)	50 mL
2 tbsp	vegetable oil	25 mL
4 tsp	chopped fresh galangal (or 1 tbsp/15 mL ground dried galangal mixed with an equal amount water)	20 mL
2 tsp	shrimp paste	10 mL
2 tsp	ground toasted coriander seeds	10 mL
2 tsp	ground toasted cumin seeds	10 mL
2 tsp	ground toasted fennel seeds	10 mL
1 1/2 tsp	salt	7 mL
1 tsp	grated kaffir lime or lime zest	5 mL
1/2 tsp	freshly ground black pepper	2 mL
1/4 tsp	ground cloves	1 mL
2 tbsp	water (approx.)	25 mL

1. In blender, on high speed, blend chilies, garlic, cilantro, bay leaves, shallots, lemon grass, oil, galangal, shrimp paste, coriander seeds, cumin seed, fennel seeds, salt, lime zest, pepper and cloves to a fine paste, scraping down sides and adding water as necessary.

2. Store in the refrigerator for up to 2 weeks, or freeze in pre-measured amounts for up to 6 months (see tip, at left).

Use in any recipe that calls for Thai red curry paste, such as meat curries and satay sauce.

TIP

Each of the spices will take a different amount of time to toast properly; some will be ready in about 30 seconds, others in about 4 minutes. Watch carefully while toasting spices, as they will become bitter if over-toasted. Spices are ready when they are very fragrant and turn a few shades deeper in color.

Thai Red Curry Paste

6	whole cloves	6
3	dried bay leaves	3
1/2	whole nutmeg	1/2
4 tsp	coriander seeds	20 mL
4 tsp	cumin seeds	20 mL
1/2 tsp	anise seeds	2 mL
1/4 tsp	black peppercorns	1 mL
1/4 tsp	white peppercorns	1 mL
15	small or medium dried red chilies	15
10	fresh Thai red chilies	10
8	cloves garlic, smashed	8
1/2 cup	chopped shallots	125 mL
1/4 cup	finely chopped lemon grass (white and light green parts only)	50 mL
1/4 cup	chopped fresh cilantro roots	50 mL
2 tbsp	vegetable oil	25 mL
4 tsp	chopped fresh galangal (or 3 tsp/15 mL ground dried galangal mixed with an equal amount water)	20 mL
1 1/2 tsp	grated kaffir lime or lime zest	7 mL
2 tsp	shrimp paste	10 mL
2 tbsp	water (approx.)	25 mL

1. In a dry heavy-bottomed skillet wiped clean of any lingering oil, over medium-low heat, separately toast cloves, bay leaves, nutmeg, coriander seeds, cumin seeds, anise seeds and black and white peppercorns, shaking them around a bit for even toasting, until fragrant and slightly darkened (see tip, at left).

2. In blender, on high speed, blend toasted spices and dried chilies to a fine powder. Add fresh Thai chilies, garlic, shallots, lemon grass, cilantro roots, oil, galangal, lime zest and shrimp paste; blend to a fine paste, scraping down sides and adding water as necessary.

3. Store in the refrigerator for up to 2 weeks, or freeze in pre-measured amounts for up to 6 months (see tip, page 80).

*Use this southern
Thai curry paste in
shrimp, fish and
vegetable curries.*

TIP

Cassia bark is
also known as Asian
cinnamon. It is
available at Chinese,
Southeast Asian and
Indian grocers.
Each of the spices
will take a different
amount of time to
toast properly; some
will be ready in about
30 seconds, others in
about 4 minutes.
Watch carefully while
toasting spices, as
they will become
bitter if over-toasted.
Spices are ready when
they are very fragrant
and turn a few shades
deeper in color.

Thai Massaman Curry Paste

10	large dried Thai or Chinese red chilies (or 8 dried New Mexico red chilies)	10
6	whole cloves	6
4	cardamom pods	4
2	small sticks cassia bark (or 1 stick cinnamon)	2
¼	whole nutmeg	¼
4 tsp	coriander seeds	20 mL
1 tbsp	cumin seeds	15 mL
1 tbsp	fennel seeds	15 mL
3 tbsp	dry-roasted peanuts	45 mL
4	cloves garlic, smashed	4
1	red onion, chopped	1
2 tbsp	finely chopped lemon grass (white and light green parts only)	25 mL
2 tbsp	peanut or vegetable oil	25 mL
1 tbsp	chopped galangal root (or 2 tsp/10 mL ground dried galangal mixed with an equal amount water)	15 mL
2 tsp	chopped gingerroot	10 mL
2 tbsp	water (approx.)	25 mL

1. In a dry heavy-bottomed skillet wiped clean of any
lingering oil, over medium-low heat, separately toast
chilies, cloves, cardamom, cassia bark, nutmeg,
coriander seeds, cumin seeds and fennel seeds, shaking
them around a bit for even toasting, until fragrant and
slightly darkened (see tip, at left).

2. In blender, on high speed, blend toasted spices and
peanuts to a fine powder. Add garlic, onion, lemon grass,
oil, galangal and ginger; blend to a fine paste, scraping
down sides and adding water as necessary.

3. Store in the refrigerator for up to 2 weeks, or freeze
in pre-measured amounts for up to 6 months (see tip,
page 80).

Soups

Basic Blender Vegetable Soup

2 cups	blanched vegetables	500 mL
4 cups	chicken or vegetable stock, divided	1 L
	Salt and freshly ground black pepper	

1. In blender, on high speed, purée vegetables with 1 cup (250 mL) of the stock.

2. Transfer to a large saucepan with remaining 3 cups (750 mL) stock. Season to taste with salt and pepper; bring to a boil over medium-high heat. Reduce heat and simmer for 2 minutes. Ladle into bowls.

Variation

For cream soup, add $1/4$ to $1/2$ cup (50 to 125 mL) whipping (35%) cream after soup has come to a boil and heat until simmering.

Celery and Pea Soup

4	stalks celery, chopped	4
2½ cups	chicken stock	625 mL
1	onion, chopped	1
¼ tsp	salt	1 mL
2½ cups	fresh or frozen peas	625 mL
2 tbsp	butter or whipping (35%) cream	25 mL
¼ tsp	freshly ground white pepper	1 mL
4 tsp	chopped celery leaves	20 mL

1. In a large saucepan, bring stock to boil over high heat. Add celery, onion and salt. Cover, reduce heat to low and simmer until vegetables are tender, about 10 minutes. Uncover, add peas and cook until tender, about 2 minutes. Add butter and pepper, increase heat and return to a boil.

2. Transfer to blender in batches and purée on high speed.

3. Pour into warmed bowls and garnish with celery leaves.

Jerusalem artichokes, or sunchokes, are a delicious root vegetable native to North America. Because of their rich artichoke-like flavor, they need few additions to make a wonderful soup. They pair naturally with butter and cream. The soup is well worth the trouble of peeling the gnarled roots.

TIPS

You can also serve the soup chilled: just replace the butter with an equal amount of olive oil. Add lemon juice to blender. Refrigerate puréed soup until chilled and stir in chilled whipping cream just before serving.

Garnish with chopped chives or chopped fresh parsley, if desired.

Jerusalem Artichoke Soup

2 tbsp	butter	25 mL
1	white onion, chopped	1
1 lb	Jerusalem artichokes, peeled and sliced	500 g
2 cups	chicken stock	500 mL
1 cup	water	250 mL
1/2 tsp	salt	2 mL
1/4 tsp	freshly ground black pepper	1 mL
Pinch	ground mace or nutmeg	Pinch
2 tsp	freshly squeezed lemon juice	10 mL
1/2 cup	whipping (35%) cream	125 mL

1. In a large saucepan, melt butter over medium-high heat. Add onion and cook, stirring, for 3 to 4 minutes, or until soft. Add Jerusalem artichokes and cook, stirring, until very lightly browned, about 2 minutes. Add stock, water, salt, pepper and mace; bring to a boil. Cover, reduce heat to low and simmer until artichokes are very tender, about 30 minutes.

2. Transfer to blender in batches and purée on high speed.

3. Return purée to saucepan, add lemon juice and bring back to a simmer over medium heat. Add whipping cream and simmer until heated through. Ladle into bowls.

Rich and creamy avocados make a wonderful base for this summer soup.

Chilled Avocado Soup

Garnish

1	tomato, peeled and diced	1
1 tbsp	chopped chives	15 mL
2 tsp	freshly squeezed lime or lemon juice	10 mL
1/4 tsp	cayenne pepper	1 mL
Pinch	salt	Pinch

Soup

2 cups	chilled defatted chicken stock	500 mL
1/2 cup	chopped sweet onion	125 mL
1/4 tsp	ground cumin	1 mL
1/4 tsp	salt	1 mL
Pinch	freshly ground white pepper	Pinch
Dash	hot pepper sauce	Dash
2	avocados, halved, pitted and peeled	2
1/2 cup	chilled whipping (35%) cream, table (18%) cream or sour cream	125 mL

1. *Prepare the garnish:* In a small bowl, mix together tomato, chives, lime juice, cayenne and salt; cover and chill for at least 2 hours or for up to 2 days.

2. *Prepare the soup:* In blender, on high speed, purée stock, onion, cumin, salt, pepper and hot pepper sauce. Add avocado and purée on high speed. On low speed, blend in cream.

3. Ladle soup into bowls and garnish with tomato mixture.

Variation

Chilled Avocado and Basil Soup: Replace whipping (35%) cream with 1/3 cup (75 mL) extra-virgin olive oil, increase lemon juice in garnish to 4 tsp (20 mL) and top with 12 shredded basil leaves.

This rich and hearty soup can be topped with shredded tortillas, grated cheese, diced cherry tomatoes, pickled jalapeños or chopped avocado.

TIPS

Quick-soak method for beans: In a large saucepan, bring beans and water to a boil for 3 minutes. Remove from heat, cover and soak for 1 hour. Drain and discard cooking liquid.

Dried beans have a much richer flavor and firmer texture than those from cans, but for convenience, you can substitute two 19-oz (540 mL) cans, drained and rinsed. Simmer for just 20 minutes, or until vegetables are tender and flavors meld.

Black Bean Soup

2 cups	dried black beans	500 mL
1 tbsp	vegetable oil	15 mL
4	cloves garlic, minced	4
1	jalapeño pepper, seeded and minced	1
1	bay leaf	1
½ cup	chopped peeled carrots	125 mL
½ cup	chopped celery	125 mL
½ cup	chopped onion	125 mL
1 tbsp	dried oregano	15 mL
½ tsp	salt	2 mL
½ tsp	freshly ground black pepper	2 mL
2 tsp	ground cumin	10 mL
4 cups	chicken stock	1 L
4 cups	water	1 L
½ cup	sour cream	125 mL
1 tsp	salt	5 mL
½ cup	prepared salsa	125 mL
2	green onions, thinly sliced	2

1. Place beans in a large bowl and cover with at least 2 inches (5 cm) water. Let soak overnight, then drain beans and discard soaking liquid.

2. In a large saucepan, heat oil over medium-high heat. Add garlic, jalapeño, bay leaf, carrots, celery, onion, oregano, salt and pepper; cook, stirring, until vegetables are soft, about 8 minutes. Add cumin and cook, stirring, for 2 minutes, until fragrant. Stir in chicken stock, water and beans; bring to a boil. Cover, reduce heat and simmer until beans are very tender, about 1 hour. Let cool.

3. With a slotted spoon, remove about 2 cups (500 mL) of the cooked beans and other solids from the soup. Transfer to blender and purée on high speed with 1 cup (250 mL) warm water. Stir back into soup. Simmer gently until heated through, about 5 minutes.

4. In a small bowl, stir together sour cream and salt.

5. Ladle soup into bowls, top with sour cream and salsa, and sprinkle with green onions.

*Beet greens, besides
being a delicious
vegetable, are one of
the highest sources
of dietary potassium.*

TIP

Toast caraway seeds
in a skillet over
medium-low heat
until fragrant and
lightly toasted, about
1 minute.

Blender Beet Borscht

4½ cups	water	1.125 L
½ cup	dry white wine	125 mL
1	small onion, chopped	1
1 tsp	salt	5 mL
1½ lbs	beets, peeled and quartered	750 g
3 cups	shredded beet greens	750 mL
½ cup	sour cream	125 mL
1 tsp	lightly toasted caraway seeds	5 mL

1. In a large saucepan, bring water, wine, onion and salt to a boil over medium-high heat. Add beets and cook until tender, about 45 minutes.

2. Transfer to blender in batches, and purée on high speed.

3. Return purée to saucepan and simmer until heated through.

4. Meanwhile, in a another large saucepan of boiling salted water, boil beet greens, if using, until tender, about 4 minutes. Drain and add to beet mixture.

5. Ladle into bowls, garnish with sour cream and sprinkle with caraway seeds.

Variation

Cold Blender Beet Borscht: Prepare through Step 4 and chill. Stir in 1 cup (250 mL) diced cucumber, omit caraway seeds, and garnish with sour cream topped with 4 tsp (20 mL) chopped fresh dill.

This rich recipe elevates a simple soup to a gourmet's delight. Use the freshest and sweetest carrots you can find. The cooked cucumbers add a delicate touch.

Cream of Carrot Soup

4	green onions	4
2 tbsp	butter	25 mL
4 cups	sliced peeled carrots	1 L
1/4 tsp	freshly ground white pepper	1 mL
2	field cucumbers (or 1 large English cucumber), peeled, seeded and chopped	2
1/3 cup	long-grain white rice	75 mL
1 1/2 cups	water	375 mL
1/2 tsp	salt	2 mL
2 cups	chicken stock, divided	500 mL
1/3 cup	whipping (35%) cream	75 mL
2 tbsp	chopped fresh chervil or minced fresh parsley	25 mL

1. Chop white part of the onions. Thinly slice 2 tbsp (25 mL) of the green part and set aside separately. Reserve any remaining green part for another use.

2. In a large saucepan, melt butter over medium-low heat; add carrots, white part of onions and pepper. Cook, stirring occasionally, until carrots are soft but not browned, about 10 minutes.

3. Stir in cucumbers, rice and water; increase heat and bring to a boil. Cover, reduce heat to low and simmer until rice is extremely soft and almost falling apart, about 40 minutes.

4. Transfer to blender in batches with 1 cup (125 mL) of the stock and purée on high speed.

5. Return purée to saucepan, stir in the remaining 1 cup (125 mL) stock and bring to a boil over medium-high heat. Reduce heat and simmer for 5 minutes. Stir in whipping cream and bring back to a simmer over medium-low heat; stir in reserved green part of onions.

6. Ladle into bowls and garnish with chervil.

Cauliflower and cheese are a match made in heaven.

Cauliflower and Cheese Soup

1	head cauliflower, coarsely chopped	1
1	white onion, quartered	1
⅔ cup	cubed Gruyère, aged Gouda or extra-old Cheddar cheese	150 mL
2 tbsp	butter	25 mL
¼ cup	whipping (35%) cream or sour cream	50 mL
Pinch	ground nutmeg	Pinch
Pinch	cayenne pepper	Pinch
Pinch	freshly ground white pepper	Pinch
2½ cups	chicken or vegetable stock	625 mL
2 tbsp	chopped chives or fresh parsley	25 mL

1. In a large saucepan of boiling salted water, cook cauliflower and onion until very tender, about 10 minutes. Drain, reserving ½ cup (125 mL) cooking water.

2. Transfer cauliflower, onion and reserved cooking water to blender and add Gruyère, butter, whipping cream, nutmeg, cayenne and pepper. Purée on high speed.

3. Return purée to saucepan, stir in stock and bring to a boil over medium-high heat. Reduce heat and simmer, stirring, for 2 minutes.

4. Ladle into bowls and garnish with chives.

The subtle flavor of cauliflower is enriched by the complex spice mixture of curry powder — especially if you use a fresh homemade mixture (see Malay Curry Powder, page 78) — and the soup is made extra rich by the addition of egg yolks.

Curried Cauliflower Soup

1	head cauliflower, coarsely chopped	1
2 tbsp	butter	25 mL
2	cloves garlic, minced	2
1	onion, chopped	1
2 tsp	grated gingerroot	10 mL
1/3 cup	chopped fresh cilantro, divided	75 mL
4 tsp	curry powder or curry paste	20 mL
1/4 tsp	turmeric	1 mL
1/2 tsp	salt	2 mL
Pinch	granulated sugar	Pinch
2 1/2 cups	chicken or vegetable stock	625 mL
2	egg yolks	2
1/2 cup	plain yogurt	125 mL
1 tsp	freshly squeezed lemon juice	5 mL

1. In a large saucepan of boiling salted water, cook cauliflower until very tender, about 10 minutes. Drain, reserving 1 cup (125 mL) cooking water; set aside. Transfer cauliflower to blender; set aside.

2. In the same saucepan, melt butter over medium heat. Add garlic, onion and ginger; cook, stirring, until onion is soft, about 6 minutes. Stir in half of the cilantro, curry powder, turmeric, salt and sugar; cook, stirring, until very fragrant, about 1 minute. Add stock and bring to a boil. Cover, reduce heat to low and simmer for 10 minutes.

3. Transfer to blender in batches and purée on high speed.

4. Return purée to saucepan, stir in reserved cooking water and bring to a boil over medium-high heat. Reduce heat and simmer for 2 minutes.

5. Meanwhile, in a small bowl, whisk together egg yolks, yogurt and lemon juice. Whisk in 1 cup (250 mL) soup. Pour into soup and simmer, stirring constantly, until very hot but not boiling and thick enough to coat the spoon, about 3 minutes.

6. Ladle into bowls and garnish with remaining cilantro.

This is the best version I know of this favorite soup. Garnish it with chopped chives, chervil or the green part of green onions, if desired.

TIP

If possible, use organic celery for fuller flavor.

Celery Soup

2	bunches green onions, chopped	2
1/4 cup	butter or extra-virgin olive oil	50 mL
1	bunch celery, chopped	1
1	potato, peeled and cubed	1
2 cups	chicken stock	500 mL
2 cups	water	500 mL
1 tsp	salt	5 mL
	Freshly ground black pepper	

1. In a large saucepan, melt butter over medium heat. Add onion, celery and potato; cook, stirring often, until celery is tender, about 10 minutes. Add stock, water and salt; bring to a boil. Cover, reduce heat and simmer for 12 to 15 minutes, or until potato begins to fall apart.

2. Transfer to blender in batches and purée on high speed.

3. Ladle into bowls and sprinkle with pepper to taste.

Celery root (celeriac) makes a rich and satisfying cold soup. At its freshest in late summer, celery root has the fragrance of celery and the texture, when cooked and blended, of very smooth potato purée. The soup is a beautiful pale green.

TIP

To serve this soup hot, return the purée to the saucepan and bring to a boil.

Cold Celery Root Soup

1 1/2 cups	cubed peeled celery root	375 mL
2 cups	chopped peeled and seeded cucumber	500 mL
1 cup	chilled water (approx.)	250 mL
1/2 cup	loosely packed fresh parsley	125 mL
1/4 cup	extra-virgin olive oil	50 mL
2 tbsp	chopped fresh basil	25 mL
3/4 tsp	salt	4 mL
1/4 tsp	freshly ground black pepper	1 mL

1. In a saucepan of boiling salted water, boil celery root until tender, about 20 minutes. Drain and chill under cold water. Drain well.

2. Transfer to blender and add cucumber, water, parsley, oil, basil, salt and pepper. Purée on high speed, thinning with more water as necessary.

3. Transfer to a large bowl, cover and chill for at least 2 hours or for up to 1 day. Ladle into bowls.

This basic yet extremely rich soup made of celery root (celeriac) is very welcome on cold days, especially after a day outside.

TIPS

To bake croutons: Toss together 1¼ cups (300 mL) cubed fresh bread, 1 tbsp (15 ml) melted butter or extra-virgin olive oil, and a generous pinch each of salt and pepper. Spread on a baking sheet and toast in a 400°F (200°C) oven or toaster oven for 8 to 10 minutes, or until crisp and golden.

To fry croutons: In a skillet, melt 4 tsp (20 mL) butter or heat 4 tsp (20 mL) extra-virgin olive oil over medium heat. Add 1¼ cup (300 mL) cubed fresh bread and sprinkle with a generous pinch each of salt and pepper. Cook, stirring frequently, until crisp and golden, about 6 minutes.

Winter Celery Root Soup

2 tbsp	butter or extra-virgin olive oil	25 mL
3	onions, chopped	3
2	celery roots, peeled and finely diced	2
2 cups	chicken stock	500 mL
1 cup	water	250 mL
½ tsp	salt	2 mL
¼ tsp	freshly ground white pepper	1 mL
Pinch	ground nutmeg	Pinch
½ cup	whipping (35%) cream	125 mL
2 tbsp	minced fresh parsley	25 mL
2 tbsp	minced celery leaves	25 mL
1 cup	freshly baked or fried croutons (see tips, at left)	250 mL

1. In a large saucepan, melt butter over medium heat. Add onions and cook, stirring, until translucent, about 3 minutes. Add celery roots, stock, water, salt, pepper and nutmeg; bring to a boil. Cover, reduce heat to low and simmer until celery root is soft and falls apart when tested with a fork, about 40 minutes.

2. Transfer to blender in batches and purée on high speed.

3. Return purée to saucepan and stir in whipping cream. Bring back to a simmer over medium-high heat, stirring constantly. Stir in parsley and celery leaves.

4. Ladle into bowls and top with croutons.

The blender allows you to give the chowder a creamy texture without the addition of milk or cream.

Non-Dairy Corn Chowder

2 tbsp	butter, olive oil or vegetable oil	25 mL
½	sweet onion, chopped	½
½	poblano pepper, chopped (or 1 jalapeño pepper, seeded and chopped)	½
4 cups	fresh or frozen corn kernels	1 L
½ tsp	grated lime zest	2 mL
1	tomato, peeled (see tip, page 63) and chopped	1
6 cups	chicken stock	1.5 L
⅓ cup	chopped fresh cilantro	75 mL
2 tbsp	freshly squeezed lime juice	25 mL
½ tsp	salt	2 mL
¼ tsp	freshly ground black pepper	1 mL

1. In a large saucepan, melt butter over medium heat. Add onion, pepper, corn and lime zest; cook, stirring, until onion is soft, about 8 minutes. Add tomato, stock, cilantro, lime juice, salt and pepper; bring to a boil. Cover, reduce heat to low and simmer for 15 minutes.

2. Transfer half the soup to blender in batches and purée on high speed.

3. Return purée to saucepan and simmer until heated through. Ladle into bowls.

Few soups could be simpler to make or more refreshing on a summer day than this one, especially if the cucumbers are from your garden. Serve with toasted baguette slices rubbed with a halved clove of garlic.

TIP

If cucumber skins are thick, you may want to peel all or half the skin off. If peeling, cut the thin slices for garnish before removing skin for a more attractive presentation.

Cold Cucumber Soup

2	large field cucumbers (or 1 large English cucumber)	2
2 cups	plain yogurt	500 mL
1 tbsp	freshly squeezed lemon juice	15 mL
1 tsp	salt	5 mL
¼ tsp	ground coriander	1 mL
Pinch	granulated sugar	Pinch
¼ cup	chilled water (approx.)	50 mL
2 tsp	chopped fresh dill or fennel fronds (or 2 tbsp/25 mL chopped chives)	10 mL
¼ tsp	freshly ground black pepper (or to taste)	1 mL

1. Trim ends from cucumbers and peel off skin, if desired (see tip, at left). Halve lengthwise and seed. Cut 12 thin slices and set aside. Chop the remaining cucumber.

2. In blender, on low speed, blend chopped cucumber, yogurt, lemon juice, salt, coriander and sugar until cucumbers are almost smooth. Thin with chilled water, if desired.

3. Ladle into bowls, garnish with cucumber slices and dill and sprinkle with pepper.

Cucumber is excellent cooked, a fact ignored by most North American cooks but quite the norm in French and Chinese cuisines. This pale green soup combines fresh and cooked cucumber and is elegant enough to serve at a dinner party.

TIPS

You can replace the lima beans with an equal amount of peeled cooked fava beans, if desired.

If pickling cucumbers are not available, substitute ¼ small English cucumber.

Cucumber and Lima Bean Soup

2	small pickling cucumbers, thinly sliced	2
1 tsp	salt, divided	5 mL
2 tbsp	extra-virgin olive oil	25 mL
3 cups	chopped, peeled and seeded cucumber	750 mL
1	sweet onion, chopped	1
2 cups	vegetable or chicken stock	500 mL
1 cup	chopped fresh cilantro	250 mL
1 cup	cooked baby lima beans	250 mL
¾ cup	half-and-half (10%) or table (18%) cream	175 mL
¼ tsp	freshly ground black pepper	1 mL
½ tsp	lightly toasted caraway or cumin seeds (see tip, page 88)	2 mL

1. In a small bowl, mix pickling cucumbers with half the salt; let stand for 15 minutes.

2. In a large saucepan, heat oil over medium-low heat. Add chopped large cucumber and onion; cook, stirring occasionally, until soft but not browned, about 7 minutes. Add stock, cilantro and remaining salt; increase heat and bring to a boil. Add lima beans. Cover, reduce heat to low and simmer until beans are tender, about 10 minutes.

3. Meanwhile, with hands, squeeze liquid out of pickling cucumbers.

4. Transfer soup to blender and purée on high speed.

5. Return purée to saucepan, stir in cream and simmer until heated through.

6. Ladle into bowls, garnish with pickling cucumber slices and sprinkle with caraway seeds.

Fennel bulbs have a remarkably subtle licorice-like flavor. This soup accentuates their delicate taste, with few added ingredients, by sautéing them in butter until they are golden brown and caramelized.

Fennel Soup

2	bulbs fennel	2
¼ cup	butter	50 mL
1	onion, quartered	1
2 tbsp	all-purpose flour	25 mL
4 cups	chicken stock	1 L
1 tsp	salt	5 mL
¼ tsp	freshly ground white pepper	1 mL
2 tbsp	sour cream or whipping (35%) cream	25 mL
2 tbsp	freshly squeezed lemon juice	25 mL

1. Remove tops from fennel bulbs, reserving 2 tbsp (25 mL) chopped fronds. Cut bulbs lengthwise into eighths.

2. In a large saucepan, melt butter over medium heat. Add fennel and onion; cook, turning pieces occasionally, until golden brown, about 20 minutes. Sprinkle with flour and cook, stirring, until flour no longer smells raw, about 2 minutes. Gradually stir in chicken stock, salt and pepper. Bring to a boil. Cover, reduce heat to low and simmer until fennel and onion are soft, about 20 minutes.

3. Transfer to blender in batches and purée on high speed.

4. Return purée to saucepan, stir in sour cream and lemon juice and simmer until heated through.

5. Ladle into bowls and sprinkle with reserved fennel fronds.

*Serve this soup with
freshly baked or fried
croutons (see tips,
page 93).*

TIPS

If you prefer a less
peppery soup, halve
the amount of black
pepper or replace
it with ¼ tsp (1 mL)
freshly ground
white pepper.

16 cloves of garlic is
about 2 large heads.

Garlic Soup

2 tbsp	extra-virgin olive oil or butter	25 mL
16	cloves garlic	16
1	white onion, chopped	1
½ tsp	freshly ground black pepper	2 mL
1	potato, peeled and diced	1
2 cups	chicken stock	500 mL
2 cups	water	500 mL
1 tsp	salt	5 mL
¼ cup	chopped fresh parsley	50 mL

1. In a large saucepan, heat oil over medium heat. Add
   garlic, onion and pepper; cook, stirring often, until
   onion is soft and garlic is lightly browned, about
   6 minutes. Add potato, stock, water and salt; bring to
   a boil. Cover, reduce heat to low and simmer until
   potatoes are soft, about 20 minutes.

2. Transfer to blender in batches and purée on high speed.

3. Return purée to saucepan and simmer until heated
   through. Stir in parsley. Ladle into bowls.

MAKES 6 SERVINGS

*This incredibly simple
soup is extremely
satisfying. Sometimes,
in cooking, as in life,
less is more. Use a
tasty white bread, such
as sourdough, and
Spanish sweet or
smoked paprika.*

TIP

16 cloves of garlic is
about 2 large heads.

Spanish Garlic Soup

3 tbsp	extra-virgin olive oil	45 mL
16	cloves garlic	16
6 cups	boiling water	1.5 L
1 tsp	salt	5 mL
12	thin slices white bread	12
½ tsp	Spanish paprika	2 mL

1. In a large saucepan, heat oil over medium heat. Add
   garlic and cook, stirring often, until garlic is golden
   brown, about 5 minutes. Add boiling water and salt.
   Cover, reduce heat to low and simmer for 30 minutes.

2. Transfer to blender in batches and purée on high speed.

3. Meanwhile, line 6 soup bowls with 2 slices bread each.

4. Return purée to saucepan and bring to a boil. Ladle soup
   over bread and sprinkle with paprika.

Bread is used as both flavoring and thickener in this Italian-style soup. If it's available, you can use black kale (also called dinosaur or dino kale) for the soup; if it is sold in small bunches, use two.

Kale and Bread Soup

4 cups	chicken or vegetable stock	1 L
2 cups	water	500 mL
4	cloves garlic, smashed	4
1	bunch kale, stemmed and shredded	1
2 cups	canned tomatoes, with juice	500 mL
3 tbsp	extra-virgin olive oil, divided	45 mL
1/4 tsp	salt	1 mL
1/4 tsp	freshly ground black pepper	1 mL
2 cups	cold water	500 mL
3 cups	cubed crustless day-old Calabrese or other Italian bread	750 mL
1 cup	chopped fresh flat-leaf parsley, divided	250 mL
1/2 cup	freshly grated Parmesan cheese	125 mL
1 tbsp	finely chopped marjoram leaves	15 mL

1. In a large saucepan, bring stock and water to a boil over high heat. Add garlic, kale, tomatoes with juice, 1 tbsp (15 mL) of the oil, salt and pepper. Cover, reduce heat to low and simmer, stirring occasionally, until kale is tender, about 20 minutes.

2. Transfer half the soup to blender in batches and purée on high speed.

3. Return purée to saucepan and bring soup back to a simmer over medium-low heat.

4. In a large bowl, drizzle cold water over bread cubes, tossing to moisten. Squeeze out excess liquid. Add to soup with 1/2 cup (125 mL) of the parsley and simmer until bread has fallen apart, about 10 minutes.

5. Stir in Parmesan, the remaining 1/2 cup (125 mL) parsley, marjoram and the remaining 2 tbsp (25 mL) oil. Ladle into bowls.

Kohlrabi, although widely grown in North America, is an underused but delicious and versatile vegetable. This soup can be served hot or cold.

TIP

If the kohlrabi has nice leaves, you can cook them like kale. If desired, shred them and cook in boiling salted water until tender, about 6 minutes. Omit dill and garnish with drained cooked leaves.

Cream of Kohlrabi Soup

2 tbsp	butter	25 mL
1	bunch kohlrabi, peeled and cut into small chunks (about 2 lbs/1 kg)	1
1	onion, chopped	1
1	potato, peeled and diced	1
¼ tsp	salt	1 mL
¼ tsp	freshly ground white pepper	1 mL
2 tbsp	all-purpose flour	25 mL
4 cups	chicken or vegetable stock	1 L
1 cup	half-and-half (10%) cream	250 mL
2 tbsp	minced chives	25 mL
2 tbsp	chopped fresh dill	25 mL

1. In a large saucepan, melt butter over medium heat. Add kohlrabi, onion, potato, salt and pepper; cook, stirring occasionally, until onion is softened, about 5 minutes. Add flour and cook, stirring, until flour no longer smells raw, about 1 minute. Slowly stir in stock; bring to a boil. Cover, reduce heat to low and simmer until vegetables are tender, about 25 minutes.

2. Transfer to blender in batches and purée on high speed. (*Make-ahead:* Cool, cover and refrigerate for up to 2 days.)

3. *To serve hot:* Return purée to saucepan and stir in cream and chives. Heat over medium heat until piping hot.

4. *To serve cold:* Let cool slightly, then refrigerate, uncovered, until cold. Stir in cream and chives.

5. Ladle into bowls and garnish with dill.

Although Swiss chard is not a particularly Swiss vegetable, Swiss Sbrinz cheese has the most complementary flavor to this Swiss-style soup. If you cannot get it, use Parmesan or another hard grating cheese — Greek kasseri cheese will be delicious. You'll be anything but disappointed with this fabulous soup.

Leek and Swiss Chard Soup

2 tbsp	butter	25 mL
2	leeks, white and light green parts only, chopped	2
2	cloves garlic, minced	2
6 cups	chicken stock	750 mL
1/3 cup	dry white wine or dry white vermouth	75 mL
1	potato, diced	1
1/2 tsp	salt	2 mL
1/4 tsp	freshly ground white pepper	1 mL
Pinch	ground nutmeg	Pinch
6 cups	Swiss chard leaves	750 mL
1/2 cup	grated Sbrinz cheese	125 mL

1. In a large saucepan, melt butter over medium heat. Add leeks and garlic; cook, stirring, until soft but not browned, about 8 minutes. Add stock, wine, potato, salt, pepper and nutmeg; bring to a boil. Cover, reduce heat to low and simmer until potatoes are completely soft, about 20 minutes. Add Swiss chard, increase heat to medium and boil until tender, about 4 minutes.

2. Transfer to blender in batches and purée on high speed.

3. Return purée to saucepan and bring to a boil over medium heat. Stir in Sbrinz. Ladle into bowls.

Welcome spring to your table with this lower-fat soup.

Green Spring Soup

1	bunch green onions	1
3 cups	chicken stock	750 mL
1 lb	potatoes, peeled and chopped	500 g
¾ tsp	salt	4 mL
¼ tsp	freshly ground black pepper	1 mL
1	bunch watercress, chopped (about 3 cups/750 mL)	1
½ cup	chopped fresh parsley	125 mL
1 cup	milk, divided	250 mL
2 tsp	cornstarch (optional)	10 mL

1. Separate white and green parts of onions and chop both.

2. In a large saucepan, bring stock, white part of onions, potatoes, salt and pepper to a boil over medium-high heat. Cover, reduce heat to low and simmer for 20 to 25 minutes, or until potatoes are tender. Add green part of onions, watercress and parsley; simmer for 1 minute.

3. Transfer to blender in batches, and purée on high speed.

4. Set aside 2 tbsp (25 mL) of the milk. Return purée to saucepan, add remaining milk and bring to a boil over medium-high heat. Reduce heat and simmer for 3 minutes.

5. If soup needs to be thickened, add cornstarch to reserved milk and stir until smooth. Stir into soup and simmer, stirring, until silky and smooth, about 2 minutes.

Wonderfully refreshing, this soup makes a terrific first course on a sultry summer evening. For a mild taste, use Boston or Romaine lettuce; for a more robust and slightly bitter flavor, use escarole or curly endive.

TIP

The size of lettuce heads varies widely. If you end up with more or less than 8 cups (2 L), the soup will still taste great.

Chilled Summer Lettuce Soup

1	field cucumber (or ½ English cucumber)	1
1 tsp	salt	5 mL
1	bunch green onions	1
	Cold water	
2 tbsp	extra-virgin olive oil	25 mL
4 cups	vegetable or chicken stock	1 L
1½ cups	cubed peeled white potatoes	375 mL
¼ tsp	freshly ground white pepper	1 mL
1	head lettuce, chopped, (about 8 cups/2 L)	1
½ cup	sour cream	125 mL

1. Halve cucumber lengthwise, seed and thinly slice. Toss with salt and let stand in a bowl for 30 minutes. Handful by handful, squeeze out as much liquid as possible. Refrigerate.

2. Meanwhile, slice white part of onions. Chop 2 tbsp (25 mL) of green part; cover with cold water and refrigerate. Reserve remaining green part for another use.

3. In a large saucepan, heat oil over medium heat. Add white part of onions and cook, stirring, until softened, about 2 minutes. Add stock, potatoes and pepper; bring to a boil. Cover, reduce heat to low and simmer until potatoes are very tender, about 20 minutes. Add lettuce and cook until tender, about 3 minutes.

4. Transfer to blender in batches and purée on high speed.

5. Transfer to a large bowl, stir in sour cream and chill for at least 4 hours or for up to 2 days.

6. Ladle into bowls and garnish with cucumber and the 2 tbsp (25 mL) green onions, drained.

MAKES 4 SERVINGS

*A friend in England
had a soup like this
every week at boarding
school, where
they seem to have a
preference for bland
white and "white-ish"
food. The mushrooms,
however, add an earthy
flavor, and I've
increased the rather
stingy amount in the
traditional soup (and
replaced margarine
with butter). It is a
great way to introduce
mushrooms to kids,
who tend to dislike
the texture of
sliced mushrooms.*

English Mushroom Soup

4 cups	white mushrooms, quartered (about 12 oz/375 g)	1 L
2 cups	water	500 mL
2 tbsp	butter	25 mL
1	onion, chopped	1
2 tbsp	all-purpose flour	25 mL
2 cups	milk	500 mL
½ tsp	salt	2 mL
⅓ cup	whipping (35%) cream	75 mL
¼ tsp	ground nutmeg	2 mL

1. In blender, on low speed, blend mushrooms and water, scraping down sides as necessary, until mushrooms are very finely chopped.

2. In a large saucepan, melt butter over medium heat. Add onion and cook, stirring often, until very soft, about 10 minutes. Sprinkle with flour and cook, stirring, for 3 to 4 minutes, or until flour is golden. Gradually add mushroom mixture, stirring, until there are no lumps. Stir in milk and salt; bring to a boil. Cover, reduce heat to low and simmer for 10 minutes. Stir in whipping cream and bring back to a simmer over medium heat.

3. Ladle into bowls and sprinkle with nutmeg.

For a more sophisticated version of mushroom soup than the previous recipe, try this one. Use dried porcini mushrooms (ceps), shiitake mushrooms, morels or other dried mushrooms.

TIP

Many supermarkets sell dried mushrooms in ½ oz (14 g) packages.

Cream of Mushroom Soup

1 oz	dried mushrooms	30 g
1 cup	warm water	250 mL
4 cups	cremini or white mushrooms, quartered (about 12 oz/375 g)	1 L
1 cup	milk	250 mL
2 tbsp	butter	25 mL
1	onion, chopped	1
1	leek, white and light green parts only, chopped	1
¼ tsp	ground nutmeg	2 mL
2 tbsp	all-purpose flour	25 mL
2 cups	chicken stock	500 mL
½ tsp	salt	2 mL
¼ tsp	dried thyme	1 mL
2 tbsp	dry sherry	25 mL
⅓ cup	whipping (35%) cream	75 mL
2 tbsp	minced fresh parsley	25 mL

1. Soak dried mushrooms in warm water until soft, about 30 minutes. Drain, reserving soaking water. Strain water through a fine sieve or coffee filter to remove grit.

2. In blender, on low speed, blend dried and fresh mushrooms, soaking water and milk, scraping down sides as necessary, until mushrooms are very finely chopped.

3. In a large saucepan, melt butter over medium heat. Add onion, leek and nutmeg; cook, stirring often, until very soft, about 10 minutes. Sprinkle with flour and cook, stirring, until flour is golden, 3 to 4 minutes. Gradually add mushroom mixture, stirring, until there are no lumps. Stir in stock, salt and thyme; bring to a boil. Cover, reduce heat to low and simmer for 15 minutes. Add sherry and simmer, uncovered, for 2 minutes. Stir in whipping cream and simmer until heated through.

4. Ladle into bowls and sprinkle with parsley.

This is a gratifying and warming soup of simple ingredients. Make it in the autumn, when onions are juicy and sweet. My Swiss grandmother used to make an onion soup just like this, but without the help of the blender, which gives it a rich and smooth texture.

TIP

If you wish, garnish with frizzled Speck (Swiss- or German-style cured bacon) or prosciutto: Finely chop 4 thin slices and cook in 1 tbsp (15 mL) butter or oil until crisp, about 3 minutes. Drain on paper towels and sprinkle over the soup.

Swiss Cream of Onion Soup

2 tbsp	butter	25 mL
3	large onions, chopped	3
1	clove garlic, minced	1
Pinch	ground nutmeg or mace	Pinch
4 tsp	all-purpose flour	20 mL
1/3 cup	dry white wine	75 mL
4 cups	chicken or veal stock	1 L
1/2 tsp	salt	2 mL
1/4 tsp	freshly ground white or black pepper	1 mL
1/4 cup	whipping (35%) cream	50 mL
1/2 cup	grated Sbrinz or Parmesan cheese	125 mL

1. In a large saucepan, melt butter over medium heat. Add onions, garlic and nutmeg; cook, stirring often, until onions are very soft but not browned, about 10 minutes. Sprinkle with flour and cook, stirring constantly, until flour no longer smells raw, about 2 minutes. Stir in wine and cook, stirring, until almost evaporated. Gradually pour in stock, stirring, and bring to a boil. Stir in salt and pepper. Cover, reduce heat to low and simmer for 15 minutes.

2. Transfer to blender in batches and blend on low speed until smooth.

3. Return to saucepan, stir in whipping cream and simmer until heated through.

4. Ladle into bowls and serve with grated cheese.

Variation

English Cream of Onion Soup: Omit butter and garlic and substitute 1 cup (250 mL) sharp Cheddar cheese for the Sbrinz. In a large saucepan, over medium heat, cook 6 slices bacon until crispy; with tongs, remove bacon and chop. Cook onions and nutmeg in bacon fat and continue with Steps 1 to 3, adding cheese in Step 3 and stirring until melted. Sprinkle with bacon.

*Parsley is seldom
given its due as an
ingredient. Although
it is ubiquitous
as a garnish or a
sprinkling of green
flecks, it is seldom
a major flavoring
ingredient. Here it
is paired with
watercress in a rich
soup that can be
served hot or chilled.*

TIP

To serve cold: Transfer
to a large bowl after
Step 3 and chill in the
refrigerator for 2 to
4 hours.

Parsley Cream Soup

3 cups	chicken stock	750 mL
1	white onion, chopped	1
3 cups	loosely packed fresh parsley leaves, divided	750 mL
2 cups	chopped watercress	500 mL
1 tsp	salt	5 mL
1 ½ cups	whipping (35%) cream	375 mL
2	egg yolks	2
Pinch	freshly ground white pepper	Pinch
Pinch	cayenne pepper	Pinch
½ cup	finely diced peeled and seeded cucumber	125 mL

1. In a large saucepan, bring stock to a boil over high heat. Add onion, 2 cups (500 mL) of the parsley, watercress and salt. Cover, reduce heat to low and simmer for 20 minutes.

2. Strain through a sieve into blender and discard solids. Add remaining parsley, whipping cream, egg yolks, pepper and cayenne. Blend on low speed until parsley is finely chopped.

3. Return mixture to saucepan over medium-low heat. Cook, stirring constantly, without letting soup boil, until thick enough to coat the spoon, about 3 minutes.

4. Ladle into bowls and garnish with cucumber.

This garlicky soup includes parsley as an ingredient rather than as a garnish, giving it a wonderfully fresh flavor.

TIPS

Use flat-leaf parsley for fuller flavor.

If desired, drizzle a little fragrant olive oil over soup before serving.

Potato-Parsley Soup

2 tbsp	extra-virgin olive oil, divided	25 mL
8	cloves garlic, minced	8
1	onion, chopped	1
1 cup	chopped fresh parsley, divided	250 mL
¼ tsp	each salt and black pepper	1 mL
2	baking potatoes, peeled and diced	2
4 cups	chicken or vegetable stock	1 L

1. In a large saucepan, heat oil over medium heat. Add garlic, onion, ⅔ cup (150 mL) of the parsley, salt and pepper; cook, stirring, until onion is softened, about 5 minutes. Add potatoes and stock; bring to a boil. Cover, reduce heat to low and simmer until potatoes are tender, about 30 minutes.

2. Transfer to blender in batches and purée on high speed.

3. Return purée to saucepan, add the remaining parsley and simmer until heated through. Ladle into bowls.

Parsnips are like sweet white carrots — and carrots would work equally well in this soup. In autumn, you can try parsley roots instead of parsnips and garnish the soup with some minced fresh parsley.

Gingery Parsnip Soup

¼ cup	butter	50 mL
3	shallots, finely chopped	3
1 lb	parsnips, peeled and diced	500 g
3 tbsp	long-grain white rice	45 mL
4 cups	chicken or vegetable stock	1 L
1 tbsp	minced gingerroot	15 mL
3 tbsp	finely chopped chives	45 mL
¼ tsp	each salt and black pepper	1 mL

1. In a large saucepan, melt butter over medium heat. Add shallots, parsnips and rice; sauté until parsnips are tender but not browned, about 20 minutes. Stir in stock and ginger; bring to a boil. Reduce heat and simmer until rice is tender, about 15 minutes.

2. Transfer to blender in batches and purée on high speed.

3. Return purée to saucepan and add chives, salt and pepper. Simmer until heated through. Ladle into bowls.

Spring Pea Soup

There's reason to celebrate the arrival of fresh peas in late spring. Their sweetness and fresh taste is unrivaled, and peas are extremely versatile. Try this soup when the first fresh peas, green onions and lettuces appear on the market or in your garden. At other times of the year, substitute chopped snow peas, chopped sugar snap peas or frozen peas.

4	green onions	4
¾ tsp	salt	4 mL
2½ cups	water	625 mL
2½ cups	fresh peas	625 mL
2 cups	coarsely chopped lettuce leaves	500 mL
½ cup	loosely packed fresh mint leaves	125 mL
Pinch	granulated sugar	Pinch
2 tbsp	butter	25 mL

1. Separate white and green parts of onions and chop green part.

2. In a large saucepan, add salt to water; bring to a boil over high heat. Add white part of green onion and boil until tender, about 1 minute. Remove with tongs, chop into pea-size bits and set aside.

3. Add peas, lettuce, mint, sugar and green part of onions to saucepan. Reduce heat and simmer for 3 to 5 minutes, or until peas are tender.

4. Strain through a sieve into blender. Remove ¼ cup (50 mL) peas and set aside. Add remaining contents of sieve to blender, add butter and purée on high speed. (If desired, return purée to saucepan and bring back to a boil.)

5. Pour into warmed bowls and garnish with white part of onions and reserved peas.

Variation

Cold Spring Pea Soup: Increase salt by a pinch and replace butter with 2 tbsp (25 mL) whipping (35%) cream. Chill soup, white part of onions and reserved peas before serving. Garnish with 2 tbsp (25 mL) chopped fresh mint.

Arugula and peas share the same season and make excellent culinary partners. You can also make this soup with frozen peas. Serve it hot or cold.

TIP

To serve cold: Increase salt to 1 tsp (5 mL). After puréeing, chill in refrigerator for at least 4 hours or for up to 2 days.

Fresh Pea and Arugula Soup

3 cups	water	750 mL
1	white onion, chopped	1
2	cloves garlic	2
¾ tsp	salt	4 mL
Pinch	granulated sugar	Pinch
2 cups	fresh peas	500 mL
1	bunch arugula	1
2 tbsp	extra-virgin olive oil	25 mL

1. In a large saucepan, bring water to a boil over high heat. Add onion, garlic, salt and sugar. Cover, reduce heat to low and simmer until onion is tender, about 10 minutes. Uncover, add peas and simmer until tender, 3 to 5 minutes.

2. Set aside 4 leaves arugula; add remainder to pot and cook for 5 seconds.

3. Transfer to blender in batches and purée on high speed. (If desired, return purée to saucepan and bring back to a boil.)

4. Cut reserved arugula leaves into thin strips (chiffonade).

5. Pour soup into bowls, drizzle each bowl with oil and garnish with arugula chiffonade.

Variation

Fresh Pea and Watercress Soup: Replace arugula with 1 bunch watercress, reserving ¼ cup (50 mL) tender leaves for garnish. Cook watercress for 30 seconds in step 2.

This elegant, simple soup is scented with mint and coconut.

TIP

Before chopping snow peas, remove ends and strings.

Snow Pea and Cilantro Soup

4 tsp	coconut or vegetable oil	20 mL
1	white onion, chopped	1
1	potato, peeled and cubed	1
1 cup	chopped fresh cilantro	250 mL
¾ tsp	dried mint	4 mL
¼ tsp	freshly ground white pepper	1 mL
3 cups	water	750 mL
4 cups	chopped trimmed snow peas	1 L
1 tsp	salt	5 mL
½ cup	thick coconut milk	125 mL
2 tbsp	chopped fresh mint or cilantro	25 mL

1. In a large saucepan, heat oil over medium heat. Add onion and cook, stirring, until soft, about 5 minutes. Add potato, cilantro, dried mint and pepper; cook, stirring, until cilantro is wilted and fragrant, about 2 minutes. Add water and bring to a boil. Cover, reduce heat to low and simmer for 10 minutes. Add peas and salt; simmer, covered, until potatoes and peas are very tender, about 10 minutes.

2. Transfer to blender in batches and purée on high speed.

3. Return purée to saucepan, stir in coconut milk and bring to a boil over medium heat, stirring.

4. Ladle into bowls and sprinkle with fresh mint.

*Very ripe pears are
essential for bringing
out the earthiness
of parsnips. Salty
garnishes such as
sliced dry-roasted
almonds, garlic
croutons or crispy
bacon best
complement the soup's
sweet flavors.*

TIP

You can replace the
soy milk with milk
or light (5%) cream
if desired.

Pear and Parsnip Soup

1 tbsp	vegetable oil	15 mL
1	clove garlic, minced	1
3 cups	chopped peeled parsnips (about 1 lb/500 g)	750 mL
¾ cup	chopped onion	175 mL
¾ cup	chopped peeled carrots	175 mL
1 tsp	dried thyme	5 mL
¼ tsp	salt	1 mL
¼ tsp	freshly ground black pepper	1 mL
2 tbsp	all-purpose flour	25 mL
3	very ripe pears, peeled, cored and chopped	3
4 cups	chicken or vegetable stock	1 L
1 cup	plain soy milk	250 mL
	Chopped fresh parsley	

1. In a large saucepan, heat oil over medium-high heat. Add garlic, parsnips, onion, carrots, thyme, salt and pepper; cook, stirring, until vegetables are soft and slightly browned, about 8 minutes. Stir in flour and cook, stirring, until flour no longer smells raw, about 2 minutes. Add pears and stock; bring to a boil. Cover, reduce heat to low and simmer until vegetables are very tender, about 15 minutes. Stir in soy milk.

2. Transfer to blender in batches and purée on high speed.

3. Pour into clean saucepan and simmer until heated through.

4. Ladle into bowls and sprinkle with parsley.

Pepper and Tomato Soup

5	slices bacon	5
2	cloves garlic, chopped	2
1	onion, chopped	1
1	bay leaf	1
2	red bell peppers, chopped	2
1 tbsp	sherry vinegar or red wine vinegar	15 mL
2 cups	drained canned tomatoes, seeded	500 mL
2 cups	beef or chicken stock	500 mL
2 cups	water	500 mL
½ tsp	salt	2 mL
¼ tsp	dried thyme	1 mL
¼ tsp	freshly ground black pepper	1 mL
2	green onions, thinly sliced	2
¼ cup	minced fresh parsley	50 mL

1. In a large saucepan, over medium heat, fry bacon until crisp. Remove from heat. With tongs, remove bacon, leaving fat in pan. Chop bacon and set aside.

2. Return saucepan to medium heat. Add garlic, onion and bay leaf; cook, stirring often, until onion is soft, about 6 minutes. Add red peppers and vinegar; cook, stirring, for 2 minutes. Add tomatoes, stock, water, salt, thyme and pepper; bring to a boil. Add chopped bacon. Cover, reduce heat to low and simmer for 30 minutes. Remove bay leaf.

3. Transfer to blender in batches and blend on high speed until smooth.

4. Return mixture to saucepan and simmer until heated through. Stir in green onions and parsley. Ladle into bowls.

Although most modern cooks add stock, true vichyssoise is made without stock so that the true flavor of the leeks and potatoes shines through. Serve this simple French country soup hot or cold.

Vichyssoise

3 tbsp	butter	45 mL
1 lb	potatoes, peeled and chopped	500 g
1 lb	leeks, white and light green parts only, chopped (about 3)	500 g
3½ cups	water	875 mL
1 tsp	salt	5 mL
¼ tsp	freshly ground black pepper	1 mL
½ cup	whipping (35%) cream or table (18%) cream	125 mL
3 tbsp	chopped chives	45 mL

1. In a large saucepan, melt butter over medium-low heat. Add potatoes and leeks; cook, stirring often, until leeks are soft but not browned, about 12 minutes. Add water, salt and pepper; increase heat and bring to a boil. Cover, reduce heat to low and simmer until potatoes are very soft, about 20 minutes.

2. Transfer to blender in batches and purée on high speed.

3. Return purée to saucepan, stir in cream and simmer until heated through.

4. Ladle into bowls and garnish with chives.

Variation

Four-Lily Vichyssoise: Enrich traditional vichyssoise with garlic and onion for a more complex flavor. (Leeks, onions, garlic and chives are all part of the lily family, hence the name.) Add 5 cloves minced garlic and 1 chopped onion with the potatoes and leeks.

Serve with croutons made from slices of baguette brushed with melted salted butter, sprinkled with a pinch of paprika and toasted in a preheated 400°F (200°C) oven for 8 to 10 minutes, or until crisp.

Cream of Spinach Soup

2 tbsp	butter	25 mL
3	cloves garlic, chopped	3
1	white onion, chopped	1
1 tbsp	all-purpose flour	15 mL
1 tsp	salt	5 mL
1/4 tsp	freshly ground white pepper	1 mL
4 cups	chicken or vegetable stock or water	1 L
1	bunch or package (10 oz/300 g) spinach	1
1/4 cup	whipping (35%) cream	50 mL
2 tsp	freshly squeezed lemon juice	10 mL
Pinch	ground nutmeg	Pinch

1. In a large saucepan, melt butter over medium heat. Add garlic and onion; cook, stirring occasionally, until softened but not browned, about 8 minutes. Stir in flour, salt and pepper; cook, stirring, until flour no longer smells raw, about 2 minutes. Gradually whisk in stock and bring to a boil. Add spinach and cook until tender, about 4 minutes.

2. Transfer to blender in batches and purée on high speed.

3. Return purée to saucepan and stir in whipping cream, lemon juice and nutmeg; simmer until heated through. Ladle into bowls.

Variation

Rich Cream of Spinach Soup with Cheese: Whisk 2 egg yolks into the whipping cream and lemon juice. Stir into purée over medium-low heat. Cook, stirring constantly, without letting soup boil, until heated through and soup is thick enough to coat a spoon, about 3 minutes. Stir in 1/3 cup (75 mL) freshly grated Parmesan or Swiss Sbrinz cheese.

For a thick and luxurious spinach-rich soup, double the amount of spinach and add an extra pinch of salt.

Cold Spinach and Parsley Soup

4 cups	water	1 L
3	cloves garlic	3
1	white onion, chopped	1
1	stalk celery, sliced	1
1	potato, peeled and diced	1
1 tsp	salt	5 mL
1	bunch or package (10 oz/300 g) spinach	1
1 cup	chopped fresh parsley	250 mL
Pinch	cayenne pepper	Pinch
1 tbsp	freshly squeezed lemon juice	15 mL
½ cup	sour cream, whipping (35%) cream or table (18%) cream	125 mL
2 tbsp	minced chives or additional fresh parsley	25 mL

1. In a large saucepan, bring water to a boil. Add garlic, onion, celery, potato and salt. Cover, reduce heat to low and simmer until potatoes are very tender, about 15 minutes. Add spinach, parsley and cayenne; increase heat and boil until spinach is tender, about 3 minutes.

2. Transfer to blender in batches and purée on high speed. Transfer to a bowl, cover and chill for at least 4 hours or for up to 2 days.

3. Pour into bowls, garnish with a dollop of sour cream and sprinkle with chives.

Variation

Cold Swiss Chard Soup: Substitute 2 cups (500 mL) chopped Swiss chard stems for the celery and 6 cups (1.5 L) loosely packed chard leaves for the spinach and parsley.

Spinach Egg Soup

This is based on the Greek avgolemono soup, which is thickened with eggs. Enjoy it hot or cold.

TIP

To serve cold: After Step 2, let cool slightly. Refrigerate, uncovered, until cold.

4 cups	chicken stock	1 L
1/4 cup	long-grain white rice	50 mL
Pinch	salt	Pinch
Pinch	freshly ground black pepper	Pinch
3	eggs	3
3 cups	chopped fresh spinach	750 mL
1/4 cup	freshly squeezed lemon juice	50 mL

1. In a large saucepan, bring stock, rice, salt and pepper to a simmer over medium heat. Cover, reduce heat to low and simmer until rice is tender, about 15 minutes.

2. In blender, on high speed, blend eggs and spinach until thickened. Add lemon juice and pulse to blend. Ladle about 1 cup (250 mL) hot soup into blender and purée. Pour back into pan. Cook over low heat, whisking, until thick enough to lightly coat a spoon, about 1 minute. Ladle into bowls.

MAKES 4 SERVINGS

White Turnip Soup

Purple-tipped white turnips are used less often in North America than this subtly flavored root vegetable deserves. You can also make this soup with rutabaga if you prefer; just cut it into chunks.

TIP

For an attractive presentation, garnish with chopped green onion, chives or fresh parsley.

2 cups	quartered peeled white turnips	500 mL
3 cups	chicken or vegetable stock	750 mL
1/4 cup	whipping (35%) cream	50 mL
2 tbsp	butter	25 mL
1/2 tsp	salt	2 mL
1/4 tsp	ground mace	1 mL
1/4 tsp	freshly ground white pepper	1 mL
2	egg yolks	2

1. In a large saucepan, boil turnips in stock for 12 to 15 minutes, or until tender.

2. Transfer to blender and add whipping cream, butter, salt, mace and pepper; purée on high speed. Blend in egg yolks.

3. Return purée to saucepan and cook over medium-low heat, without letting soup boil, until heated through and thick, about 3 minutes. Ladle into bowls.

*This simple soup gives
winter squash its due.
Make it in the autumn
and winter, when a
warming soup is
welcome and squash
has the best flavor.
Use any winter squash,
such as butternut,
Hubbard or acorn,
or sugar pie pumpkins.
The lemon cream
makes a pretty and
tasty garnish.*

TIP

For a more
pronounced lemon
flavor, mix in $\frac{1}{4}$ tsp
(1 mL) grated lemon
zest in Step 1.

Squash or Pumpkin Soup

$\frac{1}{3}$ cup	whipping (35%) cream	75 mL
2 tbsp	freshly squeezed lemon juice	25 mL
2 tbsp	butter	25 mL
2	inner stalks celery with leaves, chopped	2
1	onion, chopped	1
1	medium potato, peeled and diced	1
1	clove garlic, smashed	1
3 cups	diced peeled winter squash or pumpkin	750 mL
$\frac{1}{2}$ tsp	salt	2 mL
$\frac{1}{4}$ tsp	freshly ground white pepper	1 mL
Pinch	cayenne pepper	Pinch
3 cups	chicken stock	750 mL
1 cup	milk	250 mL
	Freshly grated nutmeg	

1. In a small bowl, mix whipping cream and lemon juice. Set aside at room temperature.

2. In a large saucepan, melt butter over medium heat. Add celery, onion, potato and garlic; cook, stirring, until onion is soft, about 5 minutes. Stir in squash, salt, pepper and cayenne; cook, stirring, for 1 minute. Add stock, cover, reduce heat to low and simmer for 15 to 20 minutes, or until squash is very soft.

3. Transfer to blender in batches and purée on high speed.

4. Return purée to saucepan, stir in milk and simmer until heated through.

5. Ladle into bowls, spoon cream mixture on top and sprinkle with nutmeg.

Squash and Pear Soup

2 tbsp	butter	25 mL
1 to 2	hot peppers, seeded and chopped	1 to 2
1	red onion, chopped	1
2 tbsp	sliced gingerroot	25 mL
4 cups	cubed peeled butternut squash	1 L
4 cups	chicken stock	1 L
1¾ cups	cubed peeled and cored pears	425 mL
¾ tsp	rice or cider vinegar	4 mL
½ tsp	salt	2 mL
¼ tsp	freshly ground white pepper	1 mL
Pinch	ground nutmeg	Pinch
Pinch	ground cinnamon	Pinch

1. In a large saucepan, melt butter over medium-high heat. Add hot peppers, onion and ginger; cook, stirring, until onion is soft, about 3 minutes. Add squash and cook, stirring, until tender, about 8 minutes. Add stock, pears, vinegar, salt, pepper, nutmeg and cinnamon; bring to a boil. Cover, reduce heat to low and simmer for 20 minutes.

2. Transfer to blender in batches and purée on high speed.

3. Return purée to saucepan and simmer until heated through. Ladle into bowls.

This delicately flavored soup is piqued with basil oil, making a lovely restaurant-like presentation suitable for entertaining.

Fennel Tomato Soup

3	cloves garlic, minced	3
1	onion, chopped	1
1	bay leaf	1
2 cups	canned tomatoes, with juice	500 mL
2 cups	vegetable or chicken stock	500 mL
2 cups	chopped fennel bulb	500 mL
1 cup	water	250 mL
1/2 cup	dry white wine	125 mL
2 tbsp	tomato paste	25 mL
1/4 tsp	salt	1 mL
1/4 tsp	hot pepper flakes (optional)	1 mL
Pinch	granulated sugar	Pinch
2 tbsp	Fresh Basil Oil (see recipe, page 57)	25 mL

1. In a large saucepan, over high heat, combine garlic, onion, bay leaf, tomatoes with juice, stock, fennel, water, wine, tomato paste, salt, hot pepper flakes (if using) and sugar; bring to a boil. Reduce heat and simmer, partially covered, for 45 minutes. Discard bay leaf.

2. Transfer to blender in batches and purée on high speed.

3. Strain purée through a fine sieve into saucepan and simmer until heated through.

4. Ladle into bowls and drizzle with Fresh Basil Oil.

MAKES 4 SERVINGS

You need very ripe red tomatoes to make this soup, so wait until the late summer or early autumn, or use 1 large can (28 oz/ 756 mL) tomatoes, drained, preferably imported from Italy or Spain. Serve with toasted garlic croûtes made from sliced baguette (see tip, below).

TIP

To make toasted garlic croûtes: Toast slices of baguette in a 400°F (200°C) oven until crispy and golden. Rub a halved garlic clove over each piece of toast and drizzle with extra-virgin olive oil or butter (whichever you used to make the soup).

Tomato Soup with Goat Cheese

1 ½ lbs	very ripe tomatoes, peeled (see tip, page 63)	750 g
2 tbsp	extra-virgin olive oil or butter	25 mL
2	cloves garlic, minced	2
1	Spanish onion, chopped	1
1 cup	water	250 mL
1 tsp	chopped fresh thyme (or ¼ tsp/1 mL crumbled dried)	5 mL
¾ tsp	salt	4 mL
¼ tsp	freshly ground black pepper	1 mL
3 tbsp	whipping (35%) cream	45 mL
4 oz	fresh goat cheese, crumbled	125 g
2 tbsp	chopped fresh cilantro or parsley	25 mL

1. Place a sieve over a large bowl and squeeze seeds out of tomatoes; drain juice into bowl and discard seeds. Coarsely chop tomatoes.

2. In a large saucepan, heat oil over medium heat. Add garlic and onion; cook, stirring, until onion is soft, about 8 minutes. Add tomatoes and their juice, water, thyme, salt and pepper; bring to a boil. Cover, reduce heat to low and simmer for 20 minutes.

3. Transfer to blender in batches and purée on high speed.

4. Return purée to saucepan, add whipping cream and simmer until heated through.

5. Ladle into warmed bowls, top with goat cheese and sprinkle with cilantro.

On hot summer days in Spain, this soup is a wonderful refresher. Wait until the height of tomato season to make this soup, and make sure to use a fragrant extra-virgin olive oil (from Spain if possible). Many Spanish cooks would increase the amount of olive oil in the soup, but for most North American palates, the amount given here is appropriate.

TIPS

If you wish, add some fresh minced hot pepper.

Adjust the garlic to taste — 5 cloves gives a very pungent garlicky taste.

Use a good loaf of baguette or country boule for the bread cubes.

If you wish, chop about ¼ cup (50 mL) each extra tomato, pepper and cucumber to garnish the smooth and silky gazpacho.

Spanish Tomato Gazpacho

1 cup	cubed crustless white bread	250 mL
3 tbsp	water	45 mL
2 to 5	cloves garlic, smashed	2 to 5
1	4-inch (10 cm) piece cucumber, peeled and chopped	1
½ cup	chopped green bell pepper	125 mL
1½ lbs	very ripe red tomatoes, chopped	750 g
1 cup	chopped sweet onion	250 mL
¾ cup	cold water	175 mL
⅓ cup	extra-virgin olive oil	75 mL
2 tbsp	white wine vinegar or cider vinegar (approx.)	25 mL
2 tbsp	sherry vinegar	25 mL
1 tsp	salt (approx.)	5 mL
¾ tsp	sugar	4 mL

1. Sprinkle bread with 3 tbsp (45 mL) water and squeeze dry.

2. In blender, in batches, on high speed, blend bread, garlic, cucumber, pepper, tomatoes, onion, cold water, oil, white wine vinegar, sherry vinegar, salt and sugar until smooth.

3. Strain through a fine sieve into a large bowl, discarding any solids. Cover and chill for at least 2 hours or for up to 1 day.

4. Taste to see if additional salt or white wine vinegar are needed and ladle into bowls.

Spain produces the most delicious almonds in the world. North American markets generally sell only California almonds, which are good but without the intense flavor and fragrance of the Spanish variety. Even so, they make a delicious and unusual summer soup.

TIP

You can purchase blanched almonds or blanch them yourself. To blanch, boil raw shelled almonds in water for 3 minutes. Drain and chill in a bowl of cold water. Slip off skins.

Almond and Garlic Gazpacho

2	slices toasted white bread, crusts removed	2
5	cloves garlic	5
1	sprig fresh thyme	1
¾ cup	milk	175 mL
1 cup	blanched almonds	250 mL
¾ tsp	salt	4 mL
¼ tsp	freshly ground white pepper	1 mL
1	small cucumber, seeded and diced	1
2 tbsp	extra-virgin olive oil	25 mL

1. Break up toast into small pieces.

2. In a large saucepan, over medium heat, simmer garlic, thyme and milk for 5 minutes. Remove and discard thyme.

3. Transfer to blender and add toast, almonds, salt and pepper. Blend on low speed until almonds are finely chopped, then on high speed until smooth.

4. Transfer to a large bowl, cover and chill for at least 2 hours or for up to 2 days.

5. Meanwhile, in a small bowl, mix cucumber and olive oil.

6. Pour almond mixture into bowls and top with cucumber mixture.

This unusual but delicious Italian soup is very rich, so it is best served in small portions as an appetizer.

TIP

Buy fresh California walnut halves and chop them in the blender to ensure freshness. Always store walnuts and other oily nuts in the refrigerator or freezer.

Walnut and Parmesan Soup

2 tbsp	butter	25 mL
1	onion, finely chopped	1
2½ cups	vegetable or chicken stock	625 mL
1 cup	very finely chopped walnuts	250 mL
½ cup	whipping (35%) cream	125 mL
¼ tsp	freshly ground black pepper	1 mL
Pinch	salt	Pinch
1 tbsp	cornstarch	15 mL
1 tbsp	cold water	15 mL
1 cup	freshly grated Parmesan cheese	250 mL
2 tbsp	chopped fresh parsley	25 mL
	Parmesan cheese shavings (optional)	

1. In a large saucepan, over medium heat, melt butter; cook onion, stirring, until softened, about 5 minutes. Add stock, walnuts, whipping cream, pepper and salt. Bring to a simmer and cook gently, stirring occasionally, for 10 minutes.

2. Transfer half of the soup to blender, in batches, and purée on high speed. Return purée to saucepan.

3. In a small bowl, combine cornstarch and cold water. Stir into soup and cook over medium heat, stirring, until thickened. Add Parmesan and stir until smooth. Taste to see if extra salt is needed.

4. Ladle into bowls and garnish with parsley and Parmesan shavings, if using.

Cheddar Cheese Soup

MAKES 4 TO 6 SERVINGS

This extravagantly rich soup is a favorite on cold winter days. Make sure to use good-quality extra-old Cheddar cheese: 3- to 5-year-old is the best. Top with freshly baked or fried croutons if desired (see tip, page 93).

3 tbsp	butter	45 mL
2	onions, chopped	2
1	parsnip or carrot, peeled and chopped	1
1	stalk celery, chopped	1
1	leek, white and light green parts only, chopped (optional)	1
¼ cup	all-purpose flour	50 mL
½ tsp	sweet paprika	2 mL
4 cups	beef, chicken or vegetable stock	1 L
½ cup	dark beer, ale, beer or dry white wine	125 mL
¼ tsp	salt	1 mL
¼ tsp	freshly ground black pepper	1 mL
2 cups	shredded extra-old Cheddar cheese (about 8 oz/250 g)	500 mL
2 tbsp	chopped fresh parsley	25 mL

1. In a large saucepan, melt butter over medium heat. Add onions, parsnip, celery and leek, if using; cook, stirring often, until onion is golden, about 12 minutes. Stir in flour and paprika and cook, stirring, until flour no longer smells raw, about 2 minutes. Gradually stir in stock, beer, salt and pepper; bring to a boil, stirring constantly. Cover, reduce heat to low and simmer for 20 minutes.

2. Transfer to blender in batches and purée on high speed.

3. Return purée to saucepan and bring back to a simmer over medium heat. Stir in Cheddar and cook, stirring, until cheese is melted. Stir in parsley. Ladle into bowls.

For a lighter and sweeter Cheddar cheese soup than the previous recipe, try this one.

TIP

For a pretty presentation, top with 1 apple, peeled, cored and diced, fried in 1 tbsp (15 mL) butter until tender and golden.

Cheddar and Cider Soup

2 tbsp	butter	25 mL
1	large white or Spanish onion, chopped	1
1	potato, peeled and cubed	1
1/4 tsp	freshly ground black pepper	1 mL
Pinch	ground nutmeg	Pinch
Pinch	ground cloves	Pinch
2 cups	chicken or vegetable stock	500 mL
2 cups	apple cider	500 mL
1/2 tsp	salt	2 mL
1 1/2 cups	shredded extra-old Cheddar cheese (about 6 oz/175 g)	375 mL
2 tbsp	chopped chives or fresh parsley	25 mL

1. In a large saucepan, melt butter over medium heat. Add onion, potato, pepper, nutmeg and cloves; cook, stirring often, until onion is soft but not browned, about 7 minutes. Pour in stock, cider and salt; bring to a boil. Cover, reduce heat to low and simmer until potatoes begin to fall apart, about 20 minutes.

2. Transfer to blender in batches and purée on high speed.

3. Return purée to saucepan and bring back to a simmer over medium heat. Stir in Cheddar and cook, stirring, until cheese is melted, without letting soup boil. Stir in chives. Ladle into bowls.

Cheddar and Beer Soup

1/4 cup	butter	50 mL
2	cloves garlic, minced	2
1 cup	diced leeks, white and light green parts only	250 mL
1/3 cup	all-purpose flour	75 mL
3 cups	chicken stock	750 mL
2 cups	brown ale	500 mL
2 tsp	hot or Dijon mustard	10 mL
1/2 cup	whipping (35%) cream	125 mL
3 cups	shredded extra-old Cheddar cheese (about 12 oz/375 g)	750 mL
1/2 tsp	hot pepper sauce	2 mL
1/2 tsp	Worcestershire sauce	2 mL
1/4 tsp	salt	1 mL
1/4 tsp	freshly ground black pepper	1 mL

1. In a large saucepan, melt butter over medium heat. Add garlic and leeks; cook, stirring, until softened, about 5 minutes. Add flour and cook, stirring, until flour no longer smells raw, about 2 minutes. Slowly stir in chicken stock, beer and mustard. Cover, reduce heat to low and simmer for 30 minutes. Add whipping cream; increase heat and bring to a boil. Remove from heat. Whisk in Cheddar, hot pepper sauce and Worcestershire sauce.

2. Transfer to blender in batches and purée on high speed.

3. Return to saucepan and simmer, stirring constantly, without letting soup boil, until heated through. Stir in salt and pepper. Ladle into bowls.

Curried Chicken Bisque

1 tbsp	vegetable oil	15 mL
2	slices bacon, chopped	2
2	cloves garlic, minced	2
1	apple, peeled, cored and chopped	1
1	bay leaf	1
¾ cup	chopped peeled carrots	175 mL
¾ cup	chopped celery	175 mL
¾ cup	chopped onion	175 mL
1 tbsp	minced gingerroot	15 mL
½ tsp	salt	2 mL
½ tsp	freshly ground black pepper	2 mL
1 tbsp	curry powder	15 mL
Pinch	cayenne pepper	Pinch
2 tbsp	all-purpose flour	25 mL
4 cups	chicken stock	1 L
1 cup	water	250 mL
4	skinless chicken drumsticks	4
½ cup	long-grain white rice	50 mL
1 cup	half-and-half (10%) cream	250 mL
4	prunes, pitted and thinly sliced	4
2 tbsp	thinly sliced green onions	25 mL

1. In a large saucepan, heat oil over medium heat. Add bacon, garlic, apple, bay leaf, carrots, celery, onions, ginger, salt and pepper; cook, stirring, until vegetables are soft, about 8 minutes. Stir in curry powder and cayenne; cook until fragrant, about 1 minute. Add flour and cook, stirring, until flour no longer smells raw, about 2 minutes. Stir in stock, water, chicken and rice. Cover, reduce heat to low and simmer until chicken is no longer pink inside, about 20 minutes. Remove chicken to a cutting board and shred. Stir cream into soup.

2. Transfer soup to blender in batches and purée on high speed.

3. Return purée to clean saucepan and simmer until heated through.

4. Ladle bisque into bowls and sprinkle with shredded chicken, prunes and green onions.

This is a wonderful spring soup. Vegetarians can make the soup with vegetable stock and replace the prosciutto with croutons fried in butter (see tip, page 93).

Asparagus Soup with Frizzled Prosciutto

2 oz	thinly sliced prosciutto	60 g
1 tbsp	vegetable oil	15 mL
1 lb	asparagus	500 g
4 cups	chicken stock	1 L
2 cups	water	500 mL
6	cloves garlic	6
1	egg yolk	1
¼ cup	whipping (35%) cream	50 mL
¼ tsp	salt	1 mL
¼ tsp	freshly ground black pepper	1 mL

1. Slice prosciutto into thin strips. In a skillet, heat oil over medium-high heat. Add prosciutto and cook until crisp, about 3 minutes. Drain on a paper towel and set aside.

2. Snap off woody ends of asparagus. Starting 2 inches (5 cm) from the tips, using a vegetable peeler, peel stalks.

3. In a large saucepan, bring stock, water and garlic to a boil. Cover, reduce heat to low and simmer for 5 minutes. Add asparagus, cover and simmer until tender-crisp, about 3 minutes. With tongs, remove asparagus. Trim off tops, slice in half lengthwise and set aside. Chop stalks, return to saucepan and simmer for 2 minutes. Remove from heat.

4. Transfer to blender in batches and purée on high speed.

5. Return purée to saucepan and bring back to a simmer over medium heat.

6. In a small bowl, whisk together egg yolk, whipping cream, salt and pepper.

7. Remove soup from heat and whisk in egg yolk mixture. Return to heat and cook, stirring, without letting soup boil, until thick enough to coat the spoon, about 3 minutes.

8. Ladle soup into bowls and top with reserved asparagus tips and prosciutto.

This soup is full of flavor and is a great way to incorporate dark green vegetables into your diet. Serve with crusty bread.

Collard Green and Sausage Soup

1 tbsp	olive or vegetable oil	15 mL
2	smoked sausages, diced	2
8	cloves garlic	8
1	onion, chopped	1
½ tsp	ground cumin	2 mL
¼ tsp	hot pepper flakes	1 mL
Pinch	salt	Pinch
1	can (19 oz/540 mL) white beans, drained and rinsed	1
1	bunch collard greens, stemmed and shredded (about 1 lb/500 g)	1
4 cups	chicken stock	1 L
2 cups	water	500 mL

1. In a large saucepan, heat oil over medium-high heat. Add sausages and cook until golden, about 4 minutes. Remove pan from heat. With a slotted spoon, remove sausages to a bowl and set aside, leaving fat in pan.

2. Return saucepan to medium-high heat, add garlic, onion, cumin, hot pepper flakes and salt; cook, stirring, until golden, about 3 minutes. Add beans, collard greens, stock and water; bring to a boil. Cover, reduce heat to low and simmer until collard greens are tender, about 30 minutes.

3. Transfer half of the soup to blender, in batches, and purée on high speed.

4. Return purée to saucepan, add sausages and cook, stirring, until heated through, about 3 minutes. Ladle into bowls.

Chickpea and Chorizo Soup

½ cup	lightly packed fresh basil leaves, divided	125 mL
⅓ cup	vegetable oil, divided	75 mL
2	cloves garlic, minced	2
½ cup	chopped peeled carrots	125 mL
½ cup	chopped celery	125 mL
½ cup	chopped onion	125 mL
2 tsp	dried oregano	10 mL
¼ tsp	salt	1 mL
¼ tsp	freshly ground black pepper	1 mL
4 cups	chicken or vegetable stock	1 L
2 cups	cooked chickpeas (or canned, drained and rinsed)	500 mL
1 cup	water	250 mL
¼ cup	half-and-half (10%) cream	50 mL
6 oz	chorizo sausage, sliced	175 g

1. Finely shred four basil leaves for garnish; set aside.

2. In blender, on high speed, blend remaining basil and 3 tbsp (45 mL) of the vegetable oil until smooth. Strain oil through a fine sieve and set aside, discarding solids.

2. In a large saucepan, heat 1 tbsp (15 mL) of the remaining vegetable oil over medium-high heat. Add garlic, carrots, celery, onion, oregano, salt and pepper; cook, stirring, until vegetables are soft, about 8 minutes. Stir in chicken stock, chickpeas and water; bring to a boil. Cover, reduce heat to low and simmer until vegetables are tender, about 20 minutes. Stir in cream.

3. Transfer 2 cups (500 mL) of the soup to blender and purée on high speed. Stir back into soup.

4. Meanwhile, in a skillet, heat the remaining 1 tbsp (15 mL) oil over medium-high heat. Add chorizo and cook for 3 to 5 minutes, or until well-browned and cooked through. Add to soup and bring to a simmer.

5. Ladle soup into bowls, drizzle with basil oil and sprinkle with shredded basil.

Smoked fish lovers will adore this uncomplicated soup.

Smoked Haddock Soup

2	potatoes, peeled and cubed	2
1	onion, chopped	1
1	leek, white and light green parts only, chopped	1
1	stalk celery, chopped	1
8 oz	smoked haddock or cod, skin on	250 g
2 cups	water	250 mL
2½ cups	milk	625 mL
¼ tsp	freshly ground white pepper	1 mL
2 tbsp	butter	25 mL
2 tsp	freshly squeezed lemon juice	10 mL
2 tbsp	minced fresh parsley	25 mL

1. In a large saucepan, bring potatoes, onion, leek, celery, fish and water to a boil. Cover, reduce heat to low and simmer until vegetables are tender, about 20 minutes. With a slotted spoon, remove fish. Pick off skin, remove any bones and discard. Return fish to saucepan and stir to break up fish. Add milk and pepper; increase heat and bring to a boil. Cover, reduce heat to low and simmer for 3 minutes.

2. Transfer to blender in batches and purée on high speed.

3. Return purée to saucepan and simmer until heated through. Stir in butter and lemon juice. When butter is melted, stir in parsley. Ladle into bowls.

This delicately flavored soup will help introduce children to the pleasures of eating fish, and it makes a wonderful starter when you are entertaining guests.

TIP

For an elegant presentation in the French tradition, garnish with 1 cup (250 mL) boiled small shrimp, small chunks of cooked lobster or crab, or ½ cup (125 mL) julienned sliced smoked salmon.

Cream of Sole Soup

2 tbsp	butter	25 mL
1	onion, chopped	1
1	clove garlic, minced	1
¼ cup	chopped fresh parsley	50 mL
2 tbsp	all-purpose flour	25 mL
3 cups	fish or chicken stock or milk	750 mL
1 tsp	salt	5 mL
¼ tsp	freshly ground white or black pepper	1 mL
1 lb	sole fillets (skin removed), sliced	500 g
⅓ cup	whipping (35%) cream	75 mL

1. In a large saucepan, melt butter over medium-low heat. Add onion and garlic; cook, stirring often, until onions are soft but not browned, about 12 minutes. Sprinkle with parsley and flour; cook, stirring, until flour no longer smells raw, about 2 minutes. Gradually stir in stock, increase heat and bring to a boil. Cover, reduce heat to low, add salt and pepper and simmer for 10 minutes. Add fish and cook until fish flakes easily with a fork, about 3 minutes.

2. Transfer to blender in batches and purée on high speed.

3. Return purée to saucepan, stir in whipping cream, and simmer until heated through. Ladle into bowls.

Sautéed Cajun shrimp update this classic soup and make a tasty garnish, but the bisque is quite enjoyable on its own.

Cajun Shrimp Bisque

1½ lbs	medium shrimp with shells	750 g
2 tbsp	vegetable oil, divided	25 mL
3 cups	chicken or vegetable stock	750 mL
¼ cup	butter	50 mL
1	bay leaf	1
¾ cup	chopped peeled carrots	175 mL
¾ cup	chopped celery	175 mL
¾ cup	chopped onion	175 mL
¼ tsp	salt	1 mL
1 cup	white wine	250 mL
1	can (14 oz/398 mL) whole tomatoes, with juice	1
¼ cup	long-grain white rice	50 mL
½ cup	water	125 mL
1 cup	whipping (35%) cream	250 mL
1	clove garlic, minced	1
½ tsp	Cajun seasoning	2 mL

1. Peel and devein shrimp. Set aside 12 shrimp (about 4 oz/125 g).

2. In a large saucepan, heat 1 tbsp (15 mL) of the oil over medium-high heat. Add shrimp shells and cook, stirring, until shells are very pink, about 3 minutes. Add stock. Cover, reduce heat to low and simmer for 10 minutes. Strain stock and discard shells.

3. Meanwhile, in another large saucepan, melt butter over medium heat. Add bay leaf, carrots, celery, onion and salt; cook, stirring, until vegetables are very soft, about 6 minutes. Add wine and cook, stirring, until reduced by half. Stir in tomatoes with juice, rice, water and strained stock; bring to a boil. Cover, reduce heat to low and simmer for 15 to 20 minutes, or until rice is tender. Add all but reserved shrimp and cook until pink and opaque, about 5 minutes. Stir in whipping cream.

4. Transfer to blender in batches and purée on high speed.

5. Strain purée through a fine sieve into clean saucepan and simmer gently until heated through.

6. Meanwhile, in a skillet, heat remaining 1 tbsp (15 mL) oil over medium-high heat. Add reserved shrimp, garlic and Cajun seasoning; cook, stirring frequently, for 3 to 5 minutes, or until shrimp are pink and opaque.

7. Ladle bisque into bowls and garnish with Cajun shrimp.

MAKES 3 TO 6 SERVINGS

Einlauf is a simple Jewish garnish for soup broth, especially chicken soup. It's an appetizing treat for sick people and is welcome at any time for the healthy.
Sei G'sund!
(Good health!)

Einlauf

2	eggs	2
1/2 cup	water	125 mL
1/3 cup	all-purpose flour	75 mL
1/4 tsp	salt	1 mL
Pinch	ground nutmeg	Pinch
4 to 6 cups	chicken stock	1 to 1.5 L

1. In blender, on low speed, blend eggs, water, flour, salt and nutmeg until smooth.

2. In a large saucepan, bring stock to a boil. In a thin stream, pour batter into boiling stock. Reduce heat and simmer for 5 minutes. Ladle in to bowls.

This is a sophisticated and delicately flavored soup, suitable for entertaining.

TIP

Use fresh-cooked or frozen crab meat — canned crab meat will not give sufficient flavor.

Asparagus and Crab Soup

12 oz	thick asparagus	375 g
2 tbsp	butter	25 mL
1/4 cup	minced shallots	50 mL
Pinch	ground mace	Pinch
1 1/2 cups	chicken stock	375 mL
1 cup	water	250 mL
1/2 cup	clam juice	125 mL
1 cup	crab meat (see tip, at left)	250 mL
2	egg yolks	2
1/4 cup	whipping (35%) cream	50 mL
1 tsp	freshly squeezed lemon juice	5 mL
Pinch	salt	Pinch
Pinch	freshly ground black pepper	Pinch

1. Snap woody ends off asparagus. Starting 2 inches (5 cm) from tips, using a vegetable peeler, peel stalks.

2. In a large saucepan, melt butter over medium heat. Add shallots and mace; cook, stirring, until shallots are soft, about 3 minutes. Add chicken stock, water and clam juice; bring to a boil. Add asparagus. Cover, reduce heat to low and simmer until asparagus is tender-crisp, about 3 minutes. With tongs, remove asparagus. Trim off tips, slice in half lengthwise and set aside. Chop stalks, return to saucepan and simmer for 2 minutes. Remove from heat.

3. Transfer to blender in batches and purée on high speed.

4. Return purée to saucepan and bring back to a simmer over medium heat. Add crab and simmer until heated through, about 2 minutes.

5. Meanwhile, in a small bowl, whisk together egg yolks, whipping cream, lemon juice, salt and pepper. Gradually whisk in 1/2 cup (125 mL) soup. Stir back into soup and cook, stirring constantly, without letting soup boil, until soup is thick enough to lightly coat the spoon, about 3 minutes.

6. Ladle into bowls and garnish with reserved asparagus tips.

Meals

BREAKFAST

DINNER ENTRÉES

SIDE DISHES

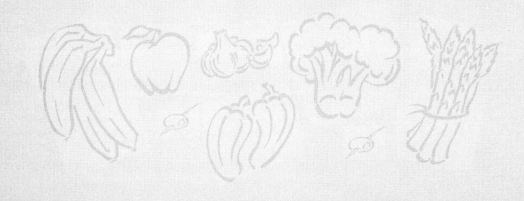

*For a healthier
alternative, replace
half the all-purpose
flour with whole wheat
flour. Serve with
maple syrup.*

Banana Pancakes

2	eggs	2
1 cup	all-purpose flour	250 mL
1 cup	milk	250 mL
3 tbsp	butter, melted, divided	45 mL
½ tsp	baking powder	2 mL
¼ tsp	salt	1 mL
2	bananas, thinly sliced	2

1. In blender, on low speed, blend eggs, flour, milk, 2 tbsp (25 mL) of the melted butter, baking powder and salt until smooth.

2. In a nonstick skillet, heat half the remaining butter over medium-high heat. Pour in batter ¼ cup (50 mL) at a time. Top each pancake with slices of banana. Cook for 2 to 3 minutes, or until bottom is golden and bubbles break on top. Turn and cook for 2 to 3 minutes, or until bottom is golden. Repeat with remaining batter, adding butter as necessary.

Banana-Soy Pancakes

1	egg	1
1 cup	soy milk	250 mL
1	banana	1
¾ cup	whole wheat flour	175 mL
¼ cup	all-purpose flour	50 mL
1 tbsp	packed brown sugar	15 mL
2 tbsp	vegetable oil, divided	25 mL
2 tsp	baking powder	10 mL
½ tsp	vanilla	2 mL

1. In blender, on low speed, blend egg, soy milk and banana until smooth. Blend in whole wheat flour, flour, sugar, 1 tbsp (15 mL) of the oil, baking powder and vanilla.

2. Heat a nonstick skillet over medium heat and brush with some of the remaining oil. Pour in batter ¼ cup (50 mL) at a time. Cook for 2 to 3 minutes, or until bottom is golden and bubbles break on top. Turn and cook for 2 to 3 minutes, or until bottom is golden. Repeat with remaining batter, adding butter as necessary.

*Yogurt adds a little
tang to pancake batter.*

Blueberry Pancakes

1	egg	1
1 cup	all-purpose flour	250 mL
1 cup	milk	250 mL
1/3 cup	plain yogurt	75 mL
2 tbsp	granulated sugar	25 mL
2 tbsp	butter, melted, divided	25 mL
2 tsp	baking powder	10 mL
1 cup	fresh blueberries	250 mL

1. In blender, on low speed, blend egg, flour, milk, yogurt, sugar, 1 tbsp (15 mL) of the butter and baking powder until smooth.

2. Heat a nonstick skillet over medium heat and brush with some of the remaining butter. Pour in batter 1/4 cup (50 mL) at a time. Sprinkle each pancake with 2 tbsp (25 mL) berries. Cook for 2 to 3 minutes, or until bottom is golden and bubbles break on top. Turn and cook for 2 to 3 minutes, or until bottom is golden. Repeat with remaining batter, adding butter as necessary.

These will be a wonderful addition to your pancake repertoire. Serve with maple syrup, applesauce or jam.

TIP

Dry cottage cheese and farmer's cheese are the same thing.

Cottage Cheese Pancakes

2	eggs	2
1 ½ cups	all-purpose flour	375 mL
¾ cup	milk	175 mL
¾ cup	dry cottage cheese	175 mL
2 tbsp	butter, melted	25 mL
½ tsp	granulated sugar	2 mL
½ tsp	baking powder	2 mL
¼ tsp	salt	1 mL
Pinch	ground cinnamon	Pinch
1 tbsp	vegetable oil	15 mL

1. In blender, on high speed, purée eggs, flour, milk, cottage cheese, butter, sugar, baking powder, salt and cinnamon.

2. In a nonstick skillet, heat half the oil over medium-high heat. Pour in batter ¼ cup (50 mL) at a time. Cook for 2 to 3 minutes, or until bottom is golden and bubbles break on top. Turn and cook for 2 to 3 minutes, or until bottom is golden. Repeat with remaining batter, adding oil as necessary.

TIP

Dry cottage cheese and farmer's cheese are the same thing.

Cottage Cheese Latkes

6	eggs	6
1 lb	dry cottage cheese	500 g
½ cup	all-purpose flour	125 mL
¼ cup	milk	50 mL
¼ tsp	salt	1 mL
¼ tsp	ground nutmeg	1 mL
Generous pinch	freshly ground white or black pepper	Generous pinch
¼ cup	confectioner's (icing) sugar	50 mL
½ tsp	ground cinnamon	2 mL
¼ cup	butter (approx.), divided	50 mL

1. In blender, on high speed, purée eggs, cottage cheese, flour, milk, salt, nutmeg and pepper. Set aside.

2. In a small bowl, mix together sugar and cinnamon. Set aside.

3. In a skillet, melt 1 tbsp (15 mL) of the butter over medium heat. Spoon in batter by generous 2 tablespoonfuls (25 mL). Cook for 2 to 3 minutes, or until bottom is lightly browned. Turn and cook for 2 to 3 minutes, or until bottom is lightly browned. Repeat with remaining batter, adding butter as necessary.

4. Sprinkle latkes with sugar-cinnamon mixture.

TIP

If you don't have buttermilk, use soured milk: add 1 tbsp (15 mL) vinegar or freshly squeezed lemon juice to 1 cup (250 mL) milk and let stand for 10 minutes.

Fluffy Buttermilk Waffles

● *Preheated waffle iron*

2	eggs, separated	2
1½ cups	buttermilk	375 mL
¼ cup	butter, melted, divided	50 mL
2 tbsp	packed brown sugar	25 mL
1 cup	all-purpose flour	250 mL
½ cup	whole wheat flour	125 mL
1 tbsp	baking powder	15 mL
¼ tsp	ground cinnamon	1 mL
¼ tsp	salt	1 mL

1. In blender, on high speed, whip egg whites until frothy. Pour into a bowl and set aside.

2. In same blender, on low speed, blend egg yolks, buttermilk, 3 tbsp (45 mL) of the butter and sugar until frothy and well combined. Add flour, whole wheat flour, baking powder, cinnamon and salt; blend, scraping down sides as necessary, until smooth. Pulse in whipped egg whites and let rest for 20 minutes.

3. Brush preheated waffle iron with some of the remaining 1 tbsp (15 mL) butter. Pour batter into center of grid, spreading to fill in. Cook for 5 to 7 minutes, until golden and no longer steaming. Remove to a warmed plate and repeat with remaining batter.

Variations

Buckwheat Waffles: Replace whole wheat flour with buckwheat flour.

Chocolate Waffles: Replace whole wheat flour with ¼ cup (50 mL) all-purpose flour and ¼ cup (50 mL) unsweetened cocoa powder, sifted.

Cornmeal Waffles: Omit brown sugar and cinnamon. Replace whole wheat flour with cornmeal and add a pinch of cayenne pepper.

Serve this classic Mexican dish with lots of rice and warm tortillas to soak up the tasty sauce.

TIP

You can replace the chicken thighs with turkey thighs. Increase the baking time by about 20 minutes.

Chicken Mole

- Preheat oven to 400°F (200°C)
- 16-cup (4 L) casserole dish with lid

1½ cups	Easy Mole Base (see recipe, opposite)	375 mL
1 cup	hot water	250 mL
1 tsp	ground coriander	5 mL
1 tsp	ground cumin	5 mL
½ tsp	salt	2 mL
½ tsp	freshly ground black pepper	2 mL
Pinch	cayenne pepper	Pinch
3 lbs	chicken thighs	1.5 kg
1 tbsp	vegetable oil	15 mL
1 tbsp	sesame seeds	15 mL
	Chopped fresh cilantro or green onion	

1. In casserole dish, combine mole base and hot water. Set aside.

2. In a small bowl, combine coriander, cumin, salt, black pepper and cayenne. Sprinkle over chicken.

3. In a nonstick skillet, heat oil over medium-high heat. In batches, brown chicken well on both sides, then add to mole sauce, stirring to coat.

4. Bake chicken, covered, in preheated oven for 40 minutes. Uncover and cook for 20 minutes longer, until juices run clear when chicken is pierced, chicken reaches an internal temperature of 170°F (75°C) and sauce is thick enough to coat a spoon. Sprinkle with sesame seeds and cilantro.

*Real mole is a day-long
event of individually
frying chilies and
spices. This very quick
version is more like
the bottled bases. Just
add chicken or turkey
and water for a rich,
flavorful dish (see
recipe, opposite).*

TIP

Makes enough for
8 servings. If you're
serving 4, freeze the
remaining sauce for
up to 3 months.

Easy Mole Base

3 tbsp	lard or vegetable oil	45 mL
3	cloves garlic	3
3 cups	chopped onion	750 mL
3 tbsp	chili powder	45 mL
2 tsp	granulated sugar	10 mL
1 tsp	ground cinnamon	5 mL
1 tsp	ground coriander	5 mL
¼ tsp	ground cloves	1 mL
2 tbsp	unsweetened cocoa powder	25 mL
2 tbsp	sesame paste or peanut butter	25 mL
1	can (14 oz/398 mL) diced tomatoes, drained	1
1 cup	water	250 mL
2 tbsp	raisins	25 mL
1 tsp	salt	5 mL

1. In a skillet, melt lard over medium-high heat. Add garlic and onions; cook, stirring, until very soft and dark golden brown, about 10 minutes.

2. Meanwhile, in a small bowl, combine chili powder, sugar, cinnamon, coriander and cloves. Stir into onions and cook, stirring frequently, until very fragrant and spices stick slightly, about 2 minutes. Stir in cocoa powder and sesame paste until sesame paste melts and is blended. Add tomatoes and water, scraping up any brown bits stuck to bottom. Add raisins and salt. Cover and bring to a boil; reduce heat to low and simmer, stirring occasionally, until very thick, about 20 minutes. Remove from heat and let cool.

3. Transfer to blender in batches and purée on high speed.

MAKES 4 SERVINGS

*Papaya or kiwi
fruit acts as a meat
tenderizer in this
well-known marinade.
Look for garam masala
and tandoori masala
in Indian markets
or in the spice section
of your supermarket,
or make your own
(see recipes, opposite).*

Chicken Tandoori

● *Rimmed baking sheet*

Tandoori Marinade

2 cups	plain yogurt	500 mL
4	cloves garlic	4
1	small onion, chopped	1
1	piece gingerroot (about 1 inch/2.5 cm), sliced	1
½ cup	chopped peeled papaya (or 1 kiwi fruit, peeled)	125 mL
¼ cup	chopped fresh cilantro	50 mL
1 tbsp	garam masala	15 mL
1 tbsp	tandoori masala	15 mL
1 tbsp	freshly squeezed lime juice	15 mL
1 tsp	salt	5 mL
2 lbs	boneless skinless chicken thighs, cut into bite-sized pieces	1 kg
	Chopped fresh cilantro, for garnish	
	Lime wedges	

1. *Prepare the Tandoori Marinade:* Place yogurt in a strainer lined with cheesecloth and let drain in the refrigerator for 1 hour. Scrape into blender (drink or discard whey) and add garlic, onion, ginger and papaya; blend on low speed until finely chopped. Add cilantro, garam masala, tandoori masala, lime juice and salt; blend until smooth.

2. In a large bowl, toss together chicken and marinade until chicken is well coated. Cover and refrigerate overnight.

3. Preheat oven to 400°F (200°C). Arrange chicken in a single layer on baking sheet. Bake in preheated oven for 25 to 30 minutes, or until coating is browned and crusty and juices run clear when chicken is pierced. Sprinkle with cilantro and serve with lime wedges.

Garam Masala

2	3-inch (7.5 cm) sticks cinnamon, smashed	2
3 tbsp	cumin seeds	45 mL
3 tbsp	coriander seeds	45 mL
1 tbsp	whole cardamom pods	15 mL
1 tbsp	whole black peppercorns	15 mL
2 tsp	whole cloves	10 mL

1. In a dry heavy-bottomed skillet wiped clean of any lingering oil, over medium-low heat, toast cinnamon, cumin seeds, coriander seeds, cardamom, peppercorns and cloves, shaking pan occasionally, for 5 to 8 minutes, or until fragrant and lightly colored.

2. Transfer to blender and grind on high speed to powder. Let cool.

3. Transfer to a sealable jar and store at a room temperature for up to 6 months.

Tandoori Masala

3 tbsp	coriander seeds	45 mL
3 tbsp	cumin seeds	45 mL
1 tbsp	cayenne pepper	15 mL
3 to 4	drops red food coloring	3 to 4

1. In a dry heavy-bottomed skillet wiped clean of any lingering oil, over medium-low heat, toast coriander seeds and cumin seeds, shaking pan occasionally, for 3 to 5 minutes, or until fragrant and lightly colored.

2. Transfer to blender and add cayenne and food coloring; grind on high speed to powder. Let cool.

3. Transfer to a sealable jar and store at room temperature for up to 6 months.

TIP

Instead of thighs, use 4 large boneless skinless chicken breasts, cut into 6 pieces each.

Chicken Tikka

12	cloves garlic, smashed	12
¼ cup	freshly squeezed lemon juice	50 mL
¼ cup	full-fat plain yogurt	50 mL
3 tbsp	coarsely chopped fresh cilantro	45 mL
3 tbsp	coarsely chopped fresh mint	45 mL
3 tbsp	chopped gingerroot	45 mL
2 tbsp	chickpea flour (optional)	25 mL
1 tsp	salt	5 mL
½ tsp	ground cardamom	2 mL
½ tsp	cayenne pepper	2 mL
½ tsp	ground cumin	2 mL
½ tsp	ground mace	2 mL
½ tsp	ground nutmeg	2 mL
½ tsp	ground turmeric	2 mL
½ tsp	freshly ground white pepper	2 mL
3 tbsp	peanut or vegetable oil	45 mL
12	boneless skinless chicken thighs (about 2 lbs/1 kg), halved	12

1. In blender, on high speed, blend garlic, lemon juice, yogurt, cilantro, mint, ginger, chickpea flour (if using), salt, cardamom, cayenne, cumin, mace, nutmeg, turmeric and white pepper to a fine paste. With motor running on low speed, through hole in top, mix in oil.

2. In a large bowl, mix chicken with paste, coating evenly. Cover and refrigerate for at least 3 hours or for up to 12 hours.

3. Preheat barbecue or broiler. Thread chicken onto skewers, leaving about 1 inch (2.5 cm) between pieces. Grill or broil on a rack, turning to cook all sides and basting once after 2 minutes, for 7 to 8 minutes, or until juices run clear when chicken is pierced. (Or roast on a rack in a 375°F (190°C) oven for 12 to 15 minutes, basting twice).

This Vietnamese marinade makes for the most delicious grilled chicken or squab. The blender makes easy work of puréeing the lemon grass, which would take at least 20 minutes of strenuous pounding if done the traditional way with a mortar and pestle.

TIPS

In Vietnam, cooks would use *mam nem* fish sauce, which is thicker and more odiferous than the widely available clear fish sauce. You can purchase *mam nem* at Chinese and Southeast Asian grocers. Regular fish sauce, however, is a wonderful substitute.

To halve chickens, remove backbone with butcher shears; cut through breast to halve. To spatchcock, remove backbone and press chicken flat.

Lemon Grass Chicken

● *Roasting pan*

6	cloves garlic	6
2	stalks lemon grass (tender white and light green parts only), finely chopped	2
1	shallot, coarsely chopped	1
3 tbsp	fish sauce	45 mL
1 tbsp	grated lime zest	15 mL
3 tbsp	freshly squeezed lime juice	45 mL
2 tsp	chopped gingerroot	10 mL
1 1/2 tsp	packed brown sugar	7 mL
1 tsp	freshly ground black pepper	5 mL
3/4 tsp	cayenne pepper	4 mL
3/4 tsp	ground fennel seed	4 mL
1/2 tsp	ground cumin	2 mL
1/4 tsp	ground cloves	1 mL
1	large chicken or 6 squabs, halved or spatchcocked	1
2 tbsp	peanut or vegetable oil	25 mL
	Lime wedges	
	Thai Cooked Chili Sauce (see recipe, page 73)	

1. In blender, on high speed, purée garlic, lemon grass, shallot, fish sauce, lime zest, lime juice and ginger. Mix in brown sugar, pepper, cayenne, fennel, cumin and cloves.

2. Rub marinade over chicken, coating evenly. Cover and refrigerate overnight or for up to 3 days.

3. Preheat oven to 375°F (190°F). Brush chicken skin with oil and place on roasting pan, skin side up. Bake in preheated oven until just pink at the leg joint, about 40 minutes for chicken, 25 minutes for squab. Finish on the grill or under the broiler on the middle rack, turning once, until skin is crispy, juices run clear when chicken is pierced and chicken reaches an internal temperature of 170°F (75°C), 5 to 10 minutes. Serve with lime wedges and hot pepper sauce, if desired.

*The key to this
wonderfully nutty
curry is toasting the
nuts and spices until
they are fragrant and
richly colored. Squeeze
lemon wedges over
steamed basmati rice
to accentuate the
nutty flavor of this
mild curry.*

Chicken and Cashew Coconut Curry

Cashew Coconut Curry Base

8 to 10	cloves garlic	8 to 10
6	whole cloves	6
3	small whole dried red chilies (or 1 tsp/5 mL dried hot pepper flakes)	3
1	cinnamon stick, broken	1
1 cup	unsweetened flaked or shredded coconut	250 mL
1/4 cup	cashews	50 mL
2 tbsp	coriander seeds	25 mL
1 tbsp	chopped gingerroot	15 mL
2 tsp	cumin seeds	10 mL
1/2 tsp	whole black peppercorns	2 mL
1 cup	warm water (approx.)	250 mL

Chicken Curry

2 lbs	boneless skinless chicken breast and/or thighs, cut into bite-sized pieces	1 kg
1 tbsp	vegetable oil	15 mL
1	small onion, chopped	1
1/2 tsp	salt	2 mL
1/2 cup	warm water	125 mL
2 cups	chicken stock	500 mL
1/2 cup	cashews	125 mL
	Fresh cilantro	
	Lemon wedges	

1. *Prepare the Cashew Coconut Curry Base:* In a dry heavy-bottomed skillet wiped clean of any lingering oil, over low heat, combine garlic, cloves, chilies, cinnamon, coconut, cashews, coriander seeds, ginger, cumin seeds and peppercorns. Toast gently, stirring frequently, for 7 to 8 minutes, until coconut is golden and spices are very fragrant. Remove to a plate and let cool. Transfer to blender, a little at a time, and blend on high speed to a smooth paste (without any large pieces of cashew or cinnamon), thinning with warm water and scraping down sides as necessary.

2. *Prepare the Chicken Curry:* In a large saucepan, heat oil over medium heat. Add onion and cook, stirring frequently, for 8 to 10 minutes, or until golden brown. Add curry base and salt; cook, stirring constantly, until dark and very fragrant, about 8 minutes (curry will stick slightly but do not let burn). Add warm water, scraping up brown bits stuck to bottom. Stir in chicken stock and bring to a boil. Add chicken and cashews; reduce heat and simmer until chicken is no longer pink inside, about 10 minutes. Sprinkle with cilantro and serve with lemon wedges.

Soaking chicken in vinegar and water is a Jamaican technique that "washes" the meat.

Oven-Roasted Jerk Chicken

● *12-cup (3 L) shallow casserole dish with lid (or foil)*

4	skinless chicken leg quarters (about 2 lbs/500 g)	4
2 cups	water	500 mL
1 tsp	white vinegar	5 mL
2	cloves garlic, minced	2
½	green bell pepper, chopped	½
¼ cup	Jerk Marinade (see recipe, opposite)	50 mL
2 tbsp	olive oil	25 mL
2 tbsp	soy sauce	25 mL
1 tsp	dried thyme leaves	5 mL
¼ tsp	freshly ground black pepper	1 mL

1. Pull away extra fat from chicken and cut at joint into thigh and drumstick, if desired. Soak in a bowl with water and vinegar for 10 minutes. Drain and pat dry.

2. Meanwhile, in casserole dish, combine garlic, green pepper, Jerk Marinade, olive oil, soy sauce, thyme and black pepper. Add chicken and toss to coat. Cover and refrigerate for at least 1 hour or for up to 1 day.

3. Preheat oven to 350°F (180°C). Bake chicken, covered, basting occasionally, for 1 hour. Uncover and roast until juices run clear when chicken is pierced and chicken reaches an internal temperature of 170°F (75°C), about 15 minutes.

MAKES 1 CUP (250 ML)

Here's a fiery tropical marinade that enlivens grilled or roasted chicken, pork and tofu. For authentic flavor, use Scotch bonnet or Habanero peppers.

TIP

Jamaican thyme, available at West Indian grocers, is more pungent than regular thyme.

Jerk Marinade

4	cloves garlic	4
3	Scotch bonnet peppers (or jalapeños), seeded	3
2 cups	chopped green onions (about 6)	500 mL
¼ cup	fresh thyme leaves (or 2 tbsp/25 mL dried)	50 mL
3 tbsp	soy sauce	45 mL
1 tbsp	ground allspice	15 mL
1 tbsp	white or cider vinegar	15 mL
1 tsp	salt	5 mL
1 tsp	freshly ground black pepper	5 mL
½ tsp	ground nutmeg	2 mL
½ tsp	ground cinnamon	2 mL

1. In blender, on high speed, blend garlic, peppers, onions, thyme, soy sauce, allspice, vinegar, salt, pepper, nutmeg and cinnamon until smooth.

2. Transfer to a sealable jar and store in the refrigerator for up to 3 months.

This basic chili is a traditional standby all over New Mexico. The high altitude and guaranteed sunshine of New Mexico's chili fields make for some of the most fragrant and tasty of all the world's hot peppers. Serve with rice or tortillas.

Beef in New Mexico Red Chili Sauce

2 tbsp	vegetable oil	25 mL
1 lb	stewing beef, venison or lamb	500 g
1	onion	1
1/3 cup	minced fresh cilantro (leaves, stems and roots)	75 mL
1 cup	New Mexico Red Chili Sauce (see recipe, opposite)	250 mL
1 cup	beef stock or water	250 mL
1/4 tsp	salt	1 mL
1/4 tsp	freshly ground black pepper	1 mL
	Water	

1. In a deep skillet or a Dutch oven, heat oil over high heat. Brown beef in two batches. Remove beef to a plate and pour off all but 1 tbsp (15 mL) fat.

2. Reduce heat to medium-high, add onion to Dutch oven and cook, stirring, until golden brown, about 6 minutes. Add cilantro and cook, stirring constantly, for 30 seconds. Add beef and stir to coat. Stir in New Mexico Red Chili Sauce, stock, salt and pepper. Cover, reduce heat to low and simmer, stirring occasionally and adding water if sauce becomes too thick, until meat is tender, about 1 1/2 hours.

This versatile sauce can be used to stew beef, lamb or venison (see recipe, opposite), top fried eggs or baked enchiladas, or add zing to any number of sauces.

TIPS

Look for unblemished dried, but still pliable, New Mexico chilies (or Mexican pasilla chilies). Frieda's® is a popular supermarket brand.

This sauce is moderately hot; adjust the number of mild and hot chilies to taste.

New Mexico Red Chili Sauce

4	dried mild New Mexico chilies or pasilla chilies	4
4	dried hot New Mexico chilies or pasilla chilies	4
3 cups	boiling water	750 mL
1 tbsp	vegetable oil	15 mL
1	onion, coarsely chopped	1
3	cloves garlic, chopped	3
¾ tsp	ground cumin	4 mL
Pinch	ground cinnamon	Pinch
1 tsp	dried oregano	5 mL
¾ tsp	salt	4 mL

1. Seed mild and hot chilies and break into pieces. Place in blender and pour in boiling water. Cover and let stand for 30 minutes.

2. Meanwhile, in a skillet, heat oil over medium heat. Add onion and cook, stirring, for 5 minutes. Add garlic, cumin and cinnamon; cook, stirring often, until onion is golden, about 5 minutes.

3. Purée chilies on high speed (if you wish, sieve any bits of skin from purée and return to blender). Add onion mixture, oregano and salt; purée on high speed.

4. Transfer to a medium saucepan and bring to a boil. Reduce heat to low and simmer, uncovered, stirring often, until the consistency of tomato sauce, about 25 minutes.

*Allowing ribs to
marinate and then
cook for a long, slow
time gives them that
finger-licking rib-fest
taste.*

Slow-Cooked Southern-Style Ribs

Southern Rib Marinade

1	small onion, chopped	1
¼ cup	vegetable oil	50 mL
2 tbsp	paprika	25 mL
2 tbsp	cider vinegar	25 mL
1 tbsp	salt	15 mL
1 tbsp	granulated sugar	15 mL
1 tbsp	packed brown sugar	15 mL
1 tbsp	ground cumin	15 mL
1 tsp	freshly ground black pepper	5 mL
½ tsp	cayenne pepper	2 mL
5 lbs	pork back ribs	2.5 kg
1 cup	barbecue sauce (optional)	250 mL

1. *Prepare the Southern Rib Marinade:* In blender, on high speed, blend onion, oil, paprika, vinegar, salt, sugar, brown sugar, cumin, pepper and cayenne to a smooth paste.

2. Trim any visible fat from ribs. If necessary, remove membrane from underside by loosening with the tip of a sharp knife and easing off. Place ribs in a large shallow glass dish. Coat ribs thoroughly with marinade, cover and refrigerate for at least 6 hours or for up to 1 day.

3. Heat 1 burner of a 2-burner barbecue or the 2 outside burners of a 3-burner barbecue to medium (or push glowing coals to one side). Place ribs on greased grill over the unlit burner (or the side without coals). Close lid and cook for 50 minutes, keeping temperature between 250°F and 300°F (120°C and 150°C), using oven thermometer if necessary. Cook, turning occasionally, until meat is tender and bones are visible at ends, about 1 hour. Baste with barbecue sauce, if using, and cook for 10 to 15 minutes, or until sticky. Cut each strip into 2 or 3 rib portions.

The chili and spice flavor of Latin barbecue is well suited to both beef and pork ribs.

Oven-Baked Ribs with Latin Spice Rub

● *Rimmed baking sheet*

Latin Spice Rib Rub

¼ cup	cumin seeds	50 mL
¼ cup	chili powder	50 mL
3	cloves garlic	3
2 tbsp	coriander seeds	25 mL
2 tsp	ground cinnamon	10 mL
1 tbsp	packed brown sugar	15 mL
1 tbsp	salt	15 mL
1 tbsp	hot pepper flakes	15 mL
1 tsp	freshly ground black pepper	5 mL
¼ cup	orange juice	50 mL
2 tbsp	vegetable oil	25 mL
5 lbs	beef ribs or pork back ribs	2.5 kg
1 cup	barbecue sauce (optional)	250 mL

1. *Prepare the Latin Spice Rib Rub:* In blender, on high speed, blend cumin seeds, chili powder, garlic, coriander seeds, cinnamon, sugar, salt pepper flakes and black pepper to powder. Add orange juice and oil; blend on low speed to a smooth paste.

2. Trim any visible fat from ribs. If necessary, remove membrane from underside of pork ribs, if using, by loosening with the tip of a sharp knife and easing off. Place ribs in large shallow glass dish. Coat ribs thoroughly with rib rub, cover and refrigerate for at least 6 hours or for up to 1 day.

3. Preheat oven to 400°F (200°C). Place ribs on baking sheet and roast in preheated oven, turning twice, until meat is tender and bones are visible at ends, about 40 minutes. Cut pork ribs, if using, into 2 or 3 rib portions. Cut beef ribs, if using, into individual ribs. Serve with barbecue sauce, if desired.

This Japanese dish, called misoyaki, yields a lovely glazed fish with an intense flavor. My favorite fish for misoyaki is sablefish (black cod) or halibut, but any thick, relatively firm fish fillet is delicious.

TIP

Miso paste is available in the Asian food sections of many large grocery stores and at all health food stores and Japanese and Korean grocers.

Miso-Marinated Grilled Fish

● *Broiling pan*

Marinade

2	small inner stalks celery with leaves, finely chopped	2
⅔ cup	light or red miso paste	150 mL
¼ cup	sake, dry sherry or Chinese rice wine	50 mL
2 tbsp	water (approx.), divided	25 mL
1 tsp	grated gingerroot	5 mL
4	green onions, trimmed	4
4	skinless fish fillets (1 ½ lb/750 g)	4
	Lemon wedges	

1. *Prepare the marinade:* In blender, on high speed, purée celery, miso, sake, 1 tbsp (15 mL) water and ginger, adding up to 1 tbsp (15 mL) more water as necessary to achieve a smooth paste.

2. Place onions in a glass or ceramic dish. Spread miso marinade evenly over fish fillets and place on top of onion. Cover and refrigerate for at least 6 hours or for up to 12 hours.

3. Preheat broiler. Scrape marinade off fish and discard. Place fish on a greased rack over broiling pan. Broil for 6 to 7 minutes, or until top is golden. Flip fish and place onions on rack; broil, turning onions once, for 6 to 7 minutes, or until onions are golden and fish flakes easily when tested with a fork. Serve with lemon wedges.

This curry paste is from Goa, on India's western coast, where they like hot and spicy foods. Use a firm-fleshed and tasty fish such as grouper or catfish, or cook a whole pomfret in the sauce, as they do in Goa.

Goan Fish Curry

Goan Fish Curry Paste

3 tbsp	tamarind paste	45 mL
½ cup	boiling water	125 mL
2 tbsp	chopped gingerroot	25 mL
2 tbsp	ground toasted coriander seeds	25 mL
2 tsp	ground toasted cumin seeds	10 mL
1 tsp	ground turmeric	5 mL
15	dried red chilies	15
3	cloves garlic, smashed	3
3 tbsp	peanut or vegetable oil	45 mL
1	small onion, chopped	1
¼ cup	chopped ripe fresh or canned tomatoes, drained	50 mL
2 cups	coconut milk	500 mL
1 tsp	salt	5 mL
4	green hot peppers, halved and seeded	4
1½ lbs	whole fish (or 1 lb/500 g fish fillets)	750 g

1. *Prepare the Goan Fish Curry Paste:* Mix tamarind paste with boiling water and smash with a fork until pulp is separated from seeds. Strain into blender, discarding seeds, and add ginger, coriander seeds, cumin seeds, turmeric, chilies and garlic. Blend on high speed to a fine paste.

2. In a skillet, heat oil over medium heat. Add onion and cook, stirring, for 6 to 8 minutes, or until golden-brown. Add curry paste and tomatoes; cook, stirring, for 2 minutes. Stir in coconut milk and salt; bring to a boil. Add hot peppers and fish, reduce heat and simmer, uncovered, until fish flakes easily when tested with a fork, about 5 minutes.

*Everybody loves fish
and chips, and this
batter is terrific.*

Beer-Battered Fish

● *Deep-fryer or heavy-bottomed pot, filled with at least
2 inches (5 cm) vegetable oil*
● *Preheat vegetable oil to 375°F (190°C)*

1	egg	1
1 cup	beer	250 mL
¾ cup	all-purpose flour, divided	175 mL
½ cup	semolina flour	125 mL
½ tsp	salt	2 mL
Pinch	cayenne pepper	Pinch
2 lbs	firm-fleshed fish, such as haddock or cod, skin removed	1 kg
1	lemon, cut into wedges	1
	Tartar Sauce (see recipe, page 56)	

1. In blender, on low speed, blend egg, beer, ½ cup
   (125 mL) of the flour, semolina flour, salt and cayenne
   pepper, scraping down sides as necessary, until smooth.
   Pour into a shallow bowl.

2. Cut fish into single-serving fillets. Working with a couple
   of pieces at a time, dredge each piece with the remaining
   ¼ cup (50 mL) all-purpose flour and dip in batter, letting
   excess drip off. Drop fish gently into hot oil and cook for
   2 to 3 minutes, or until golden-brown. Using a slotted
   spoon, transfer fish to a paper towel–lined baking sheet;
   keep warm. Repeat with remaining fish and batter. Serve
   with lemon wedges and Tartar Sauce.

*Enjoy as an appetizer
for 4 or as dinner for 2.*

Shrimp in Cilantro-Butter Sauce

- *Preheat oven to 400°F (200°C)*
- *Shallow casserole dish*

Cilantro-Butter Sauce

2	cloves garlic	2
1 cup	chopped onion	250 mL
½ cup	loosely packed fresh cilantro stems and leaves	125 mL
¼ cup	butter, melted, or extra-virgin olive oil	50 mL
2 tbsp	freshly squeezed lime juice	25 mL
Pinch	salt	Pinch
Pinch	cayenne pepper	Pinch
1 lb	shrimp, peeled and deveined	500 g
	Lime wedges (optional)	

1. *Prepare the Cilantro-Butter Sauce:* In blender, on low speed, blend garlic, onion and cilantro until finely chopped. Add butter, lime juice, salt and cayenne pepper; blend until well combined.

2. In casserole dish, toss shrimp with sauce. Bake in preheated oven, stirring once, until shrimp are pink and opaque, about 15 minutes. Serve immediately with lime wedges, if using.

Since the advent of basil pesto into North America, many cooks have developed other pestos to be used basically in the same manner as the traditional Genoese version. Here is one of my favorites.

TIP

Makes enough for 1½ lbs (750 g) pasta, or 6 servings. You can also use it for shrimp (see recipe, above) or add some to sautéed chicken or pork tenderloin.

Sautéed Shrimp with Cilantro-Almond Pesto

2 tbsp	extra-virgin olive oil	25 mL
1 lb	shrimp, peeled and deveined	500 g
¼ tsp	smoked or sweet paprika	1 mL
Pinch	ground cumin	Pinch
⅔ cup	Coriander and Almond Pesto (see recipe, below)	150 mL

1. In a medium saucepan, heat oil over medium-high heat. Add shrimp, paprika and cumin; cook, stirring, until shrimp are pink and opaque, about 3 minutes. Stir in pesto and heat through.

Cilantro-Almond Pesto

½ tsp	ground coriander seeds	2 mL
2	cloves garlic, smashed	2
1½ cups	loosely packed chopped fresh cilantro leaves and stems	375 mL
½ cup	loosely packed fresh parsley leaves	125 mL
½ cup	extra-virgin olive oil	125 mL
3 tbsp	lightly toasted blanched almonds	45 mL
1 tsp	salt	5 mL
Pinch	cayenne pepper	Pinch
⅔ cup	grated pecorino cheese	150 mL
	Hot pasta water or hot water	

1. In small skillet, over medium heat, toast coriander seeds until fragrant, about 1 minute.

2. Transfer to blender and add garlic, cilantro, parsley, oil, almonds, salt and cayenne. Purée on high speed, scraping down sides as necessary. Pulse or stir in pecorino. Add hot pasta water as necessary to thin to a sauce-like consistency.

This sauce is used to cook the huge freshwater Mekong River shrimp (or prawns) fished from Thailand to Vietnam. These lovely blue-shelled creatures have some of the sweetest meat of any shrimp available. It is, without hesitation, one of my favorite dishes from any country in the world. If the shrimp have roe, mixing it with lime juice makes for a fabulously rich-flavored sauce.

TIPS

You can buy frozen Mekong shrimp in Chinese and Southeast Asian markets or use this recipe for any shrimp or lobster.

Serve with steamed fragrant jasmine rice or baguettes to sop up the delicious sauce.

Vietnamese Mekong Shrimp

10	cloves garlic, smashed	10
10	red Thai bird chilies (or 4 hot red peppers), chopped	10
4	stalks lemon grass, thinly sliced	4
3	shallots, chopped	3
1	¾-inch (2 cm) piece gingerroot, chopped	1
½ cup	water	125 mL
3 tbsp	packed palm or light brown sugar	45 mL
3 tbsp	fish sauce	45 mL
¼ tsp	freshly ground white pepper	1 mL
⅓ cup	fish stock, clam juice or water	75 mL
2 lb	Mekong shrimp or extra-large shrimp (or one 3-lb/1.5 kg lobster), in shell	1 kg
3 tbsp	freshly squeezed lime juice	45 mL

1. In blender, on high speed, purée garlic, chilies, lemon grass, shallots, ginger, water, sugar, fish sauce and pepper.

2. Transfer to a large saucepan, add fish stock and bring to a boil. Reduce heat and simmer, uncovered, for 3 minutes.

3. With scissors, split open body of shrimp between legs. With a demitasse spoon, scoop out roe and set aside. (For lobster, ease the body out of the shell, remove the gills and discard. Spoon out any roe and the liver — tamale — and set aside.) Add shrimp (or lobster) to sauce. Simmer, covered, until opaque in thickest part, about 8 minutes for Mekong shrimp, 5 minutes for extra-large shrimp and 14 minutes for lobster.

4. Meanwhile, in a small bowl, combine lime juice and roe (and tamale, if using lobster). Stir into saucepan and heat through.

Shrimp Balchao

In Goa, vinegar is
much more commonly
used as a flavoring
and souring agent
than in other regions
of India. This fiery hot
spice-enhanced shrimp
dish can be served hot
right after making or
at room temperature
after 1 to 2 days of
"pickling" in the
refrigerator. Serve
with basmati rice.

TIP

Use small or medium
shrimp, or large
shrimp halved
lengthwise.

1/2 tsp	cumin seeds	2 mL
8	whole cloves	8
2	sticks cinnamon, smashed	2
1/2 tsp	whole black peppercorns	2 mL
10	dried red chilies	10
8	cardamom pods	8
4	cloves garlic, smashed	4
1/3 cup	coconut, cider or malt vinegar	75 mL
2 tbsp	chopped gingerroot	25 mL
1 cup	peanut or vegetable oil	250 mL
1 lb	shrimp, shelled and deveined	500 g
1	onion, chopped	1
10	curry leaves	10
1/4 cup	chopped fresh or canned tomatoes	50 mL
2 tsp	granulated sugar	10 mL
1/2 tsp	salt	2 mL

1. In a dry heavy-bottomed skillet wiped clean of any
   lingering oil, over medium-low heat, toast cumin seeds
   until fragrant and slightly darkened, about 1 minute.
   Transfer to blender. Toast cloves, cinnamon and
   peppercorns together until fragrant and peppercorns
   just begin to wiggle in skillet, about 3 minutes.
   Transfer to blender and add chilies and cardamom;
   grind on high speed to a fine powder. Add garlic,
   vinegar and ginger; purée on high speed.

2. In a skillet, heat oil over high heat. Add shrimp and
   cook until pink and opaque, about 1 1/2 minutes. Remove
   shrimp with a slotted spoon. Drain off all but 2 tbsp
   (25 mL) oil from the skillet. Reduce heat to medium,
   add onion and cook, stirring, for 6 to 8 minutes, or until
   golden brown. Add curry leaves and cook, stirring, for
   20 seconds. Stir in tomatoes and cook for 1 minute. Add
   curry paste and cook, stirring, for 2 to 3 minutes, or
   until very fragrant. Stir in sugar, salt and shrimp; cook,
   stirring, until shrimp are coated in sauce, about
   30 seconds.

This finely chopped coleslaw is for lovers of a certain international fried chicken chain's version. A modern fast-food tradition, the recipe has been in existence since the popularization of the home blender in the '50s.

TIP

For a less tart version, replace vinegar with an equal amount of freshly squeezed lemon juice.

Blender Coleslaw

2	carrots, roughly chopped	2
1	small head cabbage, roughly chopped	1
1	small green bell pepper, roughly chopped	1
½	red onion, roughly chopped	½
	Water	
1 cup	mayonnaise (store-bought or see recipe, page 54)	250 mL
⅓ cup	buttermilk	75 mL
2 tbsp	cider vinegar	25 mL
2 tsp	granulated sugar	10 mL
1 tsp	prepared mustard	5 mL
¼ tsp	salt	1 mL
¼ tsp	freshly ground black pepper	1 mL
¼ tsp	celery seed	1 mL

1. Half-fill blender with carrots, cabbage, pepper and onion; add water to within 2 inches (5 cm) of top. Blend on low speed for a few seconds, until finely chopped. Transfer to a sieve to drain. Repeat until all vegetables are chopped. Squeeze as much water out of vegetables as possible and transfer to a large bowl.

2. In blender, on low speed, blend mayonnaise, buttermilk, vinegar, sugar, mustard, salt, pepper and celery seed until well mixed. Pour over vegetables and mix well. Cover and refrigerate for at least 1 hour or for up to 3 days.

Sweet yellow tomatoes make an attractive and delicious sauce for pasta salad.

TIP

You can also make the sauce with sweet green tomatoes, such as green zebras.

Pasta Salad with Yellow Tomato Sauce

Yellow Tomato Sauce

5	ripe yellow or green tomatoes (about 1 ¼ lb/625 g), peeled and seeded (see tip, page 63)	5
2	cloves garlic, chopped	2
¾ cup	loosely packed basil leaves	175 mL
3 tbsp	extra-virgin olive oil	45 mL
1 tsp	grated lemon zest	5 mL
¾ tsp	salt	4 mL
¼ tsp	freshly ground white or black pepper	1 mL

Pasta Salad

2	stalks celery	2
1 lb	short pasta	500 g
1	yellow bell pepper	1
1 cup	cubed bocconcini or mozzarella cheese	250 mL
½ cup	chopped toasted walnuts	125 mL

1. *Prepare the Yellow Tomato Sauce:* In blender, on low speed, blend tomatoes, garlic, basil, oil, lemon zest, salt and pepper until slightly chunky. Set aside.

2. *Prepare the Pasta Salad:* In a large pot of boiling salted water, blanch celery for 20 seconds. Remove with tongs and chill under cold water. Drain, chop and set aside.

3. Add pasta to water in pot and cook according to package directions until al dente (tender to the bite). Drain, rinse under cold water and drain well.

4. Meanwhile, preheat broiler. Cut pepper in half and place on a baking sheet. Broil, skin side up, until skin is charred. Let cool, peel and cut into strips.

5. In a large bowl, combine pasta, celery, pepper, cheese, walnuts and Yellow Tomato Sauce until well mixed.

Creamed spinach makes a wonderful side dish for broiled, grilled or roasted meat and poultry and is a great way to get kids to eat spinach. For a lighter version, replace whipping cream with light sour cream.

Creamed Spinach

1 lb	spinach, trimmed	500 g
1/4 tsp	salt	1 mL
1/4 cup	whipping (35%) cream	50 mL
Pinch	ground nutmeg	Pinch
1 tbsp	butter	15 mL
3 tbsp	minced onion	45 mL

1. Rinse spinach under cold water and drain. Place spinach, with water clinging to it, in a large saucepan. Sprinkle with salt and cook, stirring once, over medium-high heat for 4 to 5 minutes, or until wilted. Drain. Transfer to blender and add whipping cream and nutmeg; blend on low speed until very finely chopped.

2. In a skillet, melt butter over medium heat. Add onion and cook until soft, about 5 minutes. Add spinach mixture and cook, stirring, until heated through.

This dish can also be made with Swiss chard leaves.

TIP

For spinach gratin, place spinach mixture in a gratin dish, sprinkle with 1/2 cup (125 mL) grated Parmesan or pecorino cheese and bake in a 400°F (200°C) oven until cheese is melted and spinach mixture is bubbling, about 15 minutes. Serve with crusty bread as a first course.

Italian Spinach

1 lb	spinach, trimmed and rinsed	500 g
1/2 cup	canned ground (crushed) tomatoes	125 mL
2 tbsp	extra-virgin olive oil	25 mL
2	cloves garlic, minced	2
2	anchovy fillets, chopped (optional)	2
1/4 tsp	salt	1 mL

1. Place spinach, with water clinging to it, in a large saucepan. Sprinkle with salt and cook, stirring once, over medium-high heat for 4 to 5 minutes, or until wilted. Drain. Transfer to blender, add tomatoes and blend on low speed until very finely chopped.

2. In a skillet, heat oil over medium heat. Add garlic, anchovies (if using) and salt (if not using anchovies, double the salt); cook, stirring, until garlic just begins to color, about 2 minutes. Add spinach mixture, bring to a simmer and cook, stirring, until heated through.

This is good side dish for roasted meats or poultry.

TIP

With Swiss chard, you get two vegetables in one. Make the purée with the leaves and cook the stems as a second vegetable. Blanch the stem in boiling salted water until tender–crisp, then sauté in olive oil with garlic.

Spiced Swiss Chard Purée

1	bunch Swiss chard (about 1 ½ lbs/750 g)	1
¼ cup	whipping (35%) cream	50 mL
1 tbsp	butter	15 mL
2	cloves garlic, minced	2
¼ tsp	salt	1 mL
¼ tsp	ground coriander	1 mL
¼ tsp	ground cumin	1 mL
¼ tsp	ground ginger	1 mL
Pinch	ground nutmeg	Pinch
Pinch	ground cloves	Pinch

1. Pull Swiss chard leaves off stems and reserve stems for another use.

2. In a large saucepan of boiling salted water, cook Swiss chard until tender, about 4 minutes. Drain, reserving ⅓ cup (75 mL) of the cooking liquid. Chill Swiss chard under cold water and drain.

3. Transfer Swiss chard to blender and add reserved cooking liquid and whipping cream; purée on high speed. Set aside.

4. In a skillet, melt butter over medium heat. Add garlic and salt; cook, stirring, until garlic is soft, about 1 minute. Add coriander, cumin, ginger, nutmeg and cloves; cook, stirring, until fragrant, about 30 seconds. Add chard purée and bring to a simmer. Reduce heat to medium-low and simmer, uncovered, stirring occasionally, until thick, about 4 minutes.

Variation

Spiced Spinach Purée: Substitute 8 cups (2 L) spinach for the Swiss chard.

Arroz Verde

1 cup	packed spinach leaves	250 mL
½ cup	packed coarsely chopped fresh cilantro	125 mL
½ tsp	salt	2 mL
1½ cups	chicken or vegetable stock or water	375 mL
1 tbsp	butter	15 mL
1 tbsp	extra-virgin olive oil or vegetable oil	15 mL
2	cloves garlic, minced	2
1	onion, finely chopped	1
2 cups	long-grain white rice	500 mL
1 cup	milk	250 mL

1. In blender, on high speed, purée spinach, cilantro, salt and stock. Set aside.

2. In a large saucepan, heat butter and oil over medium heat. Add garlic and onion; cook, stirring, until onion is soft, about 6 minutes. Stir in rice and cook, stirring, until oil is absorbed. Pour in spinach mixture and bring to a boil. Cover, reduce heat to low and simmer until liquid is absorbed, about 10 minutes. With a fork, stir in milk. Cover and cook until rice is tender, about 10 minutes. Remove from heat and let stand, covered, for 10 minutes before serving.

*Pub-style rings taste
even better when made
at home. These are
especially good with
Classic Tomato
Ketchup (see recipe,
page 48).*

Beer-Battered Onion Rings

● Deep-fryer or heavy-bottomed pot with at least 2 inches
(5 cm) vegetable oil
● Preheat vegetable oil to 375°F (190°C)

1	egg	1
1 cup	beer	250 mL
1/2 cup	all-purpose flour	125 mL
1/2 cup	semolina flour	125 mL
1/2 tsp	salt	2 mL
Pinch	cayenne pepper	Pinch
2	large sweet onions (such as Vidalia or Spanish onions)	2
	Additional salt (optional)	

1. In blender, on high speed, blend egg, beer, flour, semolina flour, salt and cayenne, scraping down sides as necessary, until smooth.

2. Cut onions into 1/4-inch (5 mm) thick slices and separate into rings. Working with a few rings at a time, dip in batter, letting excess drip off. Gently drop into hot oil and cook until golden brown, about 2 to 3 minutes. Using a slotted spoon, transfer onion rings to a baking sheet lined with paper towels; keep warm. Repeat with remaining onions and batter. Sprinkle with salt, if desired.

Yorkshire Puddings

Yorkshire pudding is a classic accompaniment to roast beef. Serve these puddings immediately, as they will deflate upon cooling.

- Preheat oven to 425°F (220°C)
- 8-cup muffin pan, well-greased

3	eggs	3
1 1/2 cups	milk	375 mL
3 tbsp	melted butter or vegetable oil	45 mL
1/2 tsp	salt	2 mL
1 1/2 cups	all-purpose flour	375 mL

1. In blender, on high speed, purée eggs, milk, butter and salt. With motor running on low speed, through hole in top, add flour and blend well. Let rest for 10 minutes.

2. Meanwhile, place prepared muffin tin in preheated oven until hot, about 5 minutes. Remove from oven and fill cups 3/4 full. Bake until golden, about 25 minutes.

**MAKES 6 SERVINGS
(12 POPOVERS)**

Popovers

Everybody loves warm popovers with a roast or stew. The batter is a cinch in a blender.

- Preheat oven to 450°F (230°C)
- 12-cup muffin pan

3	eggs	3
1 cup	milk	250 mL
1/2 tsp	salt	2 mL
Pinch	each nutmeg and cayenne	Pinch
1 cup	all-purpose flour, sifted	250 mL
6 tbsp	butter, melted	90 mL

1. In blender, on low speed, blend eggs, milk, salt, nutmeg and cayenne until frothy. With motor running, through hole in top, add flour and blend until batter is the consistency of thick cream. Let stand for 15 minutes.

2. Meanwhile, place muffin pan in preheated oven until hot, about 5 minutes. Remove from oven and pour 1 1/2 tsp (7 mL) butter into each muffin cup. Fill halfway with batter. Return to oven and bake for 20 minutes. Reduce temperature to 375°F (190°C) and bake until lightly browned, about 20 minutes.

Buckwheat crêpes are a specialty of Normandy. They are wonderful with either a savory or a sweet filling. Fill them with Creamed Spinach (see recipe, page 167) or Spiced Swiss Chard Purée (see recipe, page 168) for a side dish, or with Apple Filling (see recipe, opposite) for dessert.

TIP

Make sure you use regular buckwheat flour, sometimes sold as light buckwheat flour, not the dark variety.

**MAKES ABOUT
3 CUPS (750 ML)**

This recipe makes enough filling to fill the crêpes in the recipe above. Place filling in the center of each crêpe and fold over to make a square. Dust with icing sugar, if desired.

Buckwheat Crêpes

● *6-inch (15 cm) crêpe pan or cast-iron skillet*

⅔ cup	buckwheat flour	150 mL
½ cup	all-purpose flour	125 mL
2	eggs	2
1 cup	milk or buttermilk	250 mL
⅔ cup	water	150 mL
2 tbsp	butter, melted, divided	25 mL
½ tsp	salt	2 mL

1. In a small bowl, whisk together buckwheat flour and all-purpose flour; set aside.

2. In blender, on low speed, blend eggs, milk, water, 1 tbsp (15 mL) of the butter and salt until thoroughly blended and bubbly. With motor running, through hole in top, blend in flours until batter is smooth.

3. Heat a crêpe pan or skillet over medium-high heat and brush with some of the remaining butter. Pour a heaping ¼ cupful (50 mL) of the batter into pan, swirling to coat. Cook until bottom is golden, about 3 minutes; flip crêpe. Cook until bottom is golden, about 30 seconds. Remove to a warmed platter. Repeat with remaining batter, stacking crêpes between wax paper.

Apple Filling

4	apples, peeled, cored and sliced	4
2 tbsp	butter	25 mL
¼ cup	packed light brown sugar	50 mL
¼ tsp	ground cinnamon	1 mL
2 tbsp	Calvados or rum	25 mL

1. In a large saucepan, melt butter over medium heat. Add apples and cook, turning occasionally, until tender-crisp, about 5 minutes. Sprinkle with sugar and cinnamon. Continue cooking, turning occasionally, until apples and sauce are golden, about 5 minutes. Pour in Calvados; when heated, ignite. Let flames burn down.

Using the blender is much quicker and less messy than grating potatoes. Serve these crispy fritters with poached eggs or smoked salmon and sour cream.

Two-Tone Potato Fritters

- *Deep-fryer or heavy-bottomed pot with at least 2 inches (5 cm) vegetable oil*
- *Preheat vegetable oil to 375° F (190°C)*

3	small baking potatoes, peeled and chopped (about 3 cups/750 mL)	3
1	small sweet potato, peeled and chopped (about 1 ½ cups/375 mL)	1
1	small onion, chopped	1
	Water	
1	egg	1
1 cup	all-purpose flour	250 mL
2 tsp	baking powder	10 mL
½ tsp	salt	2 mL

1. In blender, in batches, on low speed, blend potatoes, sweet potato and onion with enough water to cover until small and chunky. Drain into a sieve, pressing out as much water as possible.

2. In a large bowl, combine potato mixture, egg, flour, baking powder and salt.

3. In batches of 2 or 3, gently drop batter by ¼ cupfuls (50 mL) into deep-fryer and fry for 2 to 3 minutes, or until golden brown with crispy edges. Turn and fry until browned, about 3 minutes. Using a slotted spoon, transfer fritters to a baking sheet lined with paper towels; keep warm. Repeat with remaining batter, heating oil as necessary between batches.

These puffy treats are much simpler to prepare than traditional soufflés. You can replace the Gruyère with any sharp cheese, such as old Cheddar, aged Gouda, Asiago or Appenzeller.

Blender Cheese Soufflés

- *Preheat oven to 350°F (180°C)*
- *Four 10-oz (300 mL) soufflé dishes or ramekins, buttered*
- *Baking sheet*

⅓ cup	freshly grated Parmesan cheese, divided	75 mL
4	eggs	4
1 cup	shredded Gruyère cheese	250 mL
½ cup	cream cheese, softened	125 mL
⅓ cup	homogenized (whole) milk	75 mL
½ tsp	dry mustard	2 mL
Pinch	salt	Pinch
Pinch	freshly ground white pepper	Pinch
2 tbsp	minced fresh parsley	25 mL
1 tbsp	minced fresh chives	15 mL

1. Sprinkle bottoms and sides of soufflé dishes with 2 tbsp (25 mL) of the Parmesan. Arrange on baking sheet.

2. In blender, on high speed, blend eggs, Gruyère, cream cheese, milk, remaining ¼ cup (50 mL) Parmesan, mustard, salt and pepper until smooth, about 30 seconds. Pulse in parsley and chives. Pour into prepared soufflé dishes. Bake in center of preheated oven until set, puffed and golden, about 30 minutes. Serve immediately.

Desserts and Sweet Sauces

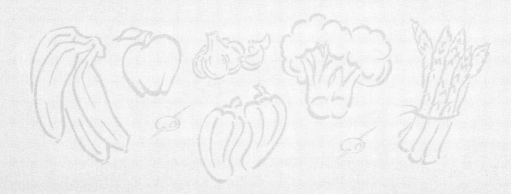

Tropical Fruit Salad

7 cups	chopped tropical fruit	1.75 L
1	mango	1
1/3 cup	liquid honey	75 mL
1 tsp	grated lime zest	5 mL
1/4 cup	freshly squeezed lime juice	50 mL
2 tbsp	shredded fresh mint (or 3/4 tsp/4 mL dried)	25 mL

Marinating the salad overnight really brings out the fresh fruit flavors. Choose an assortment of fruits with a variety of colors and shapes, such as melon, papaya, pineapple and/or star fruit.

1. Place chopped fruit in a large serving bowl. Set aside.

2. Peel the mango, cut off flesh on both sides of the pit and cut into bite-sized pieces (about 1 cup/250 mL). Add to bowl with tropical fruit.

3. Cut remaining mango flesh from around pit and place in blender. Add honey, lime zest and lime juice; purée on high speed.

4. Pour dressing over fruit salad, tossing to coat. Cover and refrigerate overnight. Sprinkle with mint before serving.

Cherry Berry Fool

1/2 cup	pitted sour cherries	125 mL
1/2 cup	fresh or frozen raspberries	125 mL
2 tbsp	raspberry or other fruit juice	25 mL
2 tbsp	liquid honey	25 mL
2 cups	whipping (35%) cream	500 mL

Red and fruity, this simple and attractive dessert will please all your guests. Use fresh, jarred or frozen sour cherries.

1. In a small saucepan, bring cherries, raspberries, juice and honey to a simmer over medium heat. Simmer until thick and jam-like, about 5 minutes. Let cool.

2. Transfer to blender and purée on high speed. Press through a fine sieve to remove seeds.

3. In the same blender, on high speed, blend whipping cream, scraping down sides as necessary, until very thick. Add cherry purée and pulse to blend.

4. Scrape into a bowl, cover with plastic wrap and refrigerate for 2 to 4 hours, until chilled, or for up to 1 day.

TIPS

To peel apricots, dunk in boiling water for 10 to 15 seconds. Chill in cold water and slip off skin.

You can use preserved apricot halves. Substitute 2 cups (500 mL) drained preserved apricot halves for the fresh apricots and reduce the sugar to ⅓ cup (75 mL). Boil for 15 minutes in Step 1.

If desired, swirl a little crème fraiche, whipping cream or sweetened sour cream into each bowl.

Apricot Dessert Soup

2 cups	water (approx.)	500 mL
1 lb	fresh apricots, peeled, halved and pitted (see tip, at left)	500 g
½ cup	granulated sugar	125 mL
1 tbsp	cornstarch	15 mL
2 tbsp	water	25 mL
½ tsp	finely grated orange zest	2 mL
¼ tsp	ground cinnamon	1 mL
Scant pinch	salt	Scant pinch
2 tbsp	apricot brandy or brandy (optional)	25 mL

1. In a large saucepan, bring the 2 cups (500 mL) water to a boil. Add apricots and sugar. Cover, reduce heat to low and simmer for 30 minutes. Transfer to blender.

2. In a small bowl, mix cornstarch and the 2 tbsp (25 mL) water until smooth. Add to blender and purée on high speed.

3. Return purée to saucepan and add orange zest, cinnamon and salt. Simmer on low heat for 20 minutes, adding additional boiling water as necessary to thin. Stir in brandy, if using, and simmer for 2 minutes. Serve hot.

Sweet Cherry Soup

¼ cup	sour cream	50 mL
2 tsp	confectioner's (icing) sugar	10 mL
1 tsp	freshly squeezed lemon juice	5 mL
½	lemon	½
2 cups + 1 tbsp	water, divided	515 mL
2½ cups	pitted cherries	625 mL
½ cup	dry red wine	125 mL
⅓ cup	granulated sugar	75 mL
¼ tsp	ground cinnamon	1 mL
2 tsp	cornstarch	10 mL
1 tbsp	Kirsch (optional)	15 mL

1. In a small bowl, combine sour cream, confectioner's sugar and lemon juice. Set aside.

2. Zest lemon with vegetable peeler and cut off white pith. Cut lemon in half, seed and chop. Place lemon zest and flesh in blender with 2 cups (500 mL) of the water and blend on high speed until very smooth.

3. Pour into a large saucepan and add cherries, wine, sugar and cinnamon; bring to a boil. Reduce heat and simmer, uncovered, for 10 minutes.

4. Mix cornstarch with the remaining 1 tbsp (15 mL) water until smooth. Stir into soup and simmer for 3 minutes, until slightly thickened.

5. Transfer to blender and purée on high speed.

6. Return purée to saucepan and simmer until heated through. Stir in Kirsch, if using.

7. *To serve hot:* Ladle into bowls and top with sour cream mixture.

8. *To serve cold:* Let cool, then refrigerate for 2 to 4 hours, until chilled. Ladle into bowls and swirl in sour cream mixture.

Madeira Strawberry Soup

4 cups	chilled hulled strawberries, divided	1 L
2 tbsp + 1 tsp	granulated sugar, divided	30 mL
Pinch	salt	Pinch
1/2 cup	chilled whipping (35%) cream	125 mL
3 tbsp	Madeira wine	45 mL

1. Slice 1 cup (250 mL) of the strawberries. In a small bowl, mix sliced strawberries with 1 tsp (5 mL) of the sugar and salt. Let stand for 5 minutes.

2. In blender, on high speed, whip cream with the remaining 2 tbsp (25 mL) sugar until thick and creamy, about 30 seconds. Add Madeira and mix on low speed. Add the remaining 3 cups (750 mL) whole strawberries and blend on low speed until smooth. With a spoon, stir in sliced strawberries. Scrape into bowls.

Melon Soup

2 cups	cubed cantaloupe	500 mL
1/3 cup	plain yogurt	75 mL
2 tbsp	liquid honey	25 mL
2 tbsp	sweet or medium-dry sherry	25 mL
1/2 tsp	vanilla	2 mL
4	sprigs fresh mint	4

1. In blender, on high speed, purée cantaloupe, yogurt, honey, sherry and vanilla.

2. Pour into bowls and refrigerate for 2 to 4 hours, until chilled, if desired. Garnish with mint.

With fresh blueberries, this is a fabulous summer dessert soup; with frozen berries, it can bring a hint of summer to the table during cooler months.

TIP

Instead of discarding the vanilla bean pods after scraping out the seeds, rinse them, pat dry and place in a sealed jar of granulated sugar to make vanilla sugar.

Cold Blueberry Soup

1	lemon	1
1 cup	dry white wine	250 mL
1/2 cup	liquid honey	125 mL
2	sprigs fresh mint	2
1	vanilla bean, split lengthwise	1
1	cinnamon stick	1
3 cups	fresh or frozen wild blueberries	750 mL
1/4 cup	whipping (35%) cream	50 mL

1. Grate zest from lemon, cut in half and juice.

2. In a large saucepan, bring lemon zest and juice, wine, honey, mint, vanilla bean halves and cinnamon to a boil. Reduce heat and simmer until slightly reduced, about 5 minutes.

3. Strain through a fine mesh sieve into clean saucepan. Scrape seeds out of vanilla beans into pan. Add blueberries, bring to a simmer and simmer for 5 minutes. Let cool.

4. Transfer to blender and pulse until almost smooth. Pour into a bowl, cover and refrigerate for 2 to 4 hours, until chilled, or for up to 2 days.

5. Pour into bowls. Drizzle whipping cream into soup and swirl in with tip of a knife.

The fruit flavors of this soup are best when served slightly chilled.

Papaya Rum Soup

3 cups	cubed, seeded and peeled papaya (about 2)	750 mL
1 cup	papaya or mango nectar	250 mL
1/4 cup	dark rum or coconut rum	50 mL
1 cup	White Chocolate Coconut Sauce (see recipe, page 208)	250 mL

1. In blender, on high speed, purée papaya, nectar and rum.

2. Pour into shallow soup bowls and refrigerate for 2 to 4 hours, until chilled, if desired. Swirl in White Chocolate Coconut Sauce, leaving soup marbled.

If you like the combination of orange and dairy (think Creamsicle) you'll love this dessert soup.

Orange Buttermilk Dessert Soup

1 1/2 cups	buttermilk	375 mL
1 1/3 cup	good-quality vanilla bean ice cream	325 mL
1 tsp	finely grated orange zest	5 mL
1 cup	freshly squeezed orange juice	250 mL
3 tbsp	granulated sugar	45 mL
	Freshly ground nutmeg	
4	thin orange slices	4

1. In blender, on high speed, purée buttermilk, ice cream, orange zest, orange juice and sugar.

2. Pour into shallow soup bowls. Sprinkle with nutmeg and float an orange slice in each bowl.

You can use any soft fruit — berries or very ripe stone fruit, such as peaches or nectarines — for this anise-flavored sorbet.

TIP

For a less icy, smoother and denser sorbet, prepare recipe through Step 3, then break mixture into small chunks and return to blender with ½ cup (125 mL) water. Pulse, scraping down sides and pushing any icy chunks down every once in a while, until smooth. Scrape into an airtight container, cover and freeze as directed.

Strawberry Anise Sorbet

● *8- or 9-inch (2 or 2.5 L) square metal baking pan*

1 cup	water	250 mL
⅓ cup	granulated sugar	75 mL
6	star anise	6
4 cups	fresh or thawed frozen strawberries	1 L
4 tsp	freshly squeezed lemon juice	20 mL

1. In a small saucepan, bring water, sugar and star anise to boil. Reduce heat and simmer until reduced to a generous ⅓ cup (75 mL), about 10 minutes.

2. Strain into blender; discard star anise. Add strawberries and lemon juice; purée on high speed.

3. Pour into a shallow metal pan, cover with plastic wrap and freeze until firm, about 4 hours.

4. Scrape the tines of a fork over the frozen mixture to create loose crystals. Scrape crystals into an airtight container, cover and freeze for at least 30 minutes or for up to 4 weeks. Scoop into chilled bowls.

*Surprise your friends
with this taste of
the tropics.*

Papaya Lemon Grass Sorbet

● *8- or 9-inch (2 or 2.5 L) square metal baking pan*

2	stalks lemon grass	2
1	long strip lemon zest	1
1 cup	water	250 mL
⅓ cup	granulated sugar	75 mL
4 cups	cubed, seeded and peeled papaya	1 L
4 tsp	freshly squeezed lemon juice	20 mL

1. Bruise lemon grass stalks with the side of a knife, then chop into 1-inch (2.5 cm) lengths.

2. In a small saucepan, bring lemon grass, lemon zest, water and sugar to a boil. Reduce heat and simmer until reduced to a generous ⅓ cup (75 mL), about 10 minutes.

3. Strain into blender; discard solids. Add papaya and lemon juice; purée on high speed.

4. Pour into a shallow metal pan, cover with plastic wrap and freeze until firm, about 4 hours.

5. Scrape the tines of a fork over the frozen mixture to create loose crystals. Scrape crystals into an airtight container, cover and freeze for at least 30 minutes or for up to 4 weeks. Scoop into chilled bowls.

Taking the time to blend this sorbet slowly, scraping down the sides of the blender and pushing down the chunks of coconut mixture, may take patience, but it results in the ultimate creamy, icy texture. Resist the temptation to add extra water — it will blend eventually.

Coconut Sorbet

● *8- or 9-inch (2 or 2.5 L) square metal baking pan*

1	can (14 oz/398 mL) coconut milk	1
1	banana	1
½ cup	sweetened flaked coconut	125 mL
¼ cup	granulated sugar	50 mL
1 tsp	grated lime zest	5 mL
2 tbsp	freshly squeezed lime juice	25 mL
1 tsp	vanilla	5 mL
⅔ cup	water	150 mL

1. In blender, on high speed, purée coconut milk, banana, coconut, sugar, lime zest, lime juice and vanilla.

2. Pour into a shallow metal pan, cover with plastic wrap and freeze until firm, about 4 hours.

3. Break mixture into small chunks and return to blender with water. Pulse, scraping down sides and pushing any icy chunks down every once in a while, until smooth.

4. Scrape into an airtight container, cover and freeze for at least 1 hour or for up to 4 weeks.

Blueberry Vanilla Sorbet

● *8- or 9-inch (2 or 2.5 L) square metal baking pan*

1	vanilla bean, split lengthwise	1
1 cup	water	250 mL
⅓ cup	granulated sugar	75 mL
4 cups	fresh or frozen wild blueberries	1 L
4 tsp	freshly squeezed lemon juice	20 mL

1. Scrape seeds from vanilla bean and place seeds and
scraped bean into a small saucepan. Add water and sugar;
bring to boil. Reduce heat and simmer until reduced to
a generous ⅓ cup (75 mL), about 10 minutes.

2. Strain into blender and add blueberries and lemon juice;
purée on high speed.

3. Pour into a shallow metal pan, cover with plastic wrap
and freeze until firm, about 4 hours.

4. Scrape a fork over the frozen mixture to create loose
crystals. Scrape into an airtight container, cover and
freeze for at least 30 minutes or for up to 4 weeks.

Peach Melba Pops

1½ cups	sliced peaches	375 mL
3 tbsp	sweetened condensed milk	45 mL
2 tsp	freshly squeezed lemon juice	10 mL
¾ cup	fresh or frozen raspberries	175 mL
2 tsp	liquid honey	10 mL

1. In blender, on high speed, purée peaches, condensed
milk and lemon juice. Scrape into a spouted container.

2. In blender, on high speed, purée raspberries and honey.
Strain through a fine sieve into a bowl.

3. Pour half of the peach mixture into 4 Popsicle molds
or small disposable cups. Spoon half of the raspberry
mixture over top. Repeat layers. Insert wooden sticks,
swirl colors together, if desired, and freeze until firm,
about 4 hours. Store for up to 1 week.

This is so easy you may never go out for ice cream again. Chop the nuts as much or as little as you like.

Butter Pecan Ice Cream

● *13- by 9-inch (3 L) metal baking pan*

3 tbsp	butter	45 mL
1 cup	pecan halves	250 mL
2 cups	whipping (35%) cream	500 mL
2 cups	half-and-half (10%) cream	500 mL
½ cup	packed brown sugar	125 mL
1 tbsp	bourbon (or 2 tsp/10 mL vanilla)	15 mL

1. In a large saucepan, melt butter over medium heat. Add pecans and cook, stirring, until nuts are lightly fried and butter starts to brown, about 5 minutes. With a slotted spoon, remove nuts and set aside.

2. To saucepan, add whipping cream, half-and-half cream, brown sugar and bourbon; bring to a boil. Reduce heat and simmer until sugar is melted, about 2 minutes. Remove from heat and let cool for 10 minutes

3. Pour cream mixture into baking pan, cover and freeze until firm, about 1 hour.

4. In blender, pulse reserved pecans until chopped to desired consistency. Remove pecans from blender and set aside.

5. In same blender, on low speed, gradually add chunks of frozen cream a few at a time, blending until smooth. When all ice cream is added and smooth and aerated, pour in pecans and pulse just to mix.

6. Return to baking pan, cover and freeze for at least 4 hours, until firm, or for up to 3 days.

Mango-Lime Semifreddo

- 9-inch (2.5 L) square metal baking pan
- 9- by 5-inch (2 L) loaf pan, lined with plastic wrap

½ cup	granulated sugar	125 mL
¼ cup	water	50 mL
2 cups	chopped peeled mangoes (about 2 large)	500 mL
1 tsp	grated lime zest	5 mL
½ cup	freshly squeezed lime juice	125 mL
1 cup	whipping (35%) cream	250 mL

1. In small saucepan, bring sugar and water to a boil. Stir until sugar is melted and clear. Set aside.

2. In blender, purée mangoes on high speed. Add lime zest, lime juice and sugar syrup; blend until well combined. Pour into baking pan and freeze until almost solid, about 1 hour.

3. In clean blender, on low speed, whip cream to soft peaks.

4. With a knife, break up frozen mango mixture. Add to blender with cream and blend on low speed until smooth and well combined.

5. Scrape into prepared loaf pan and fold plastic over to seal. Freeze for at least 4 hours, until firm, or for up to 3 days.

6. To serve, using plastic wrap, lift frozen loaf out of pan and place on cutting board. Slice into 1-inch (2.5 cm) slices.

Indian-style ice cream, or kulfi, is traditionally frozen in cone-shaped metal containers and rubbed between the hands to release. Individual-serving yogurt containers make good substitutes.

Pistachio Kulfi

● *6 kulfi or Popsicle molds or three 6-oz (175 g) yogurt containers*

4 cups	homogenized (whole) or 2% milk	1 L
4	cardamom pods, broken	4
¼ cup	granulated sugar	50 mL
¼ cup	whole almonds	50 mL
¼ cup	whole pistachios	50 mL
1½ tsp	rose water (optional)	7 mL

1. In a large saucepan, over low heat, simmer milk and cardamom until reduced to 2 cups (500 mL), about 30 minutes. Stir in sugar until dissolved.

2. Meanwhile, in blender, on high speed, chop almonds and pistachios until very fine. Sift through a sieve to remove any large pieces. Add to milk mixture with rose water, if using.

3. Pour into kulfi molds and freeze for at least 4 hours, until firm, or for up to 3 days.

This rich and chocolaty dessert takes minutes to prepare, but is elegant enough for a dinner party.

This recipe contains raw eggs. If the food safety of raw eggs is a concern for you, use the pasteurized liquid whole egg instead.

Chocolate Pots

⅔ cup	half-and-half (10%) cream	150 mL
2	eggs (or ½ cup/125 mL pasteurized liquid whole egg)	2
8 oz	bittersweet chocolate, chopped	250 g
⅓ cup	granulated sugar	75 mL
2 tbsp	brandy	25 mL

1. In a small saucepan, over medium heat, heat cream until steaming and bubbles form around edge.

2. In blender, pulse eggs, chocolate and sugar until chocolate is finely chopped. Ladle in one-quarter of the hot cream and blend on high speed for 10 seconds. Pour in remaining cream and brandy; blend until smooth.

3. Pour into demitasse or custard cups, cover and refrigerate for at least 2 hours, until set, or for up to 3 days.

Full-fat yogurt (at least 3.5%) is needed to ensure the smooth, creamy texture. You can make other flavors with any kind of frozen or fresh fruit — just adjust the sugar to taste.

Strawberry Freeze

● *9-inch (2.5 L) square metal baking pan*

2 cups	strawberries	500 mL
1/4 cup	liquid honey	50 mL
1 1/2 cups	vanilla-flavored yogurt	375 mL
1/3 cup	whipping (35%) cream	75 mL

1. In blender, on high speed, purée strawberries and honey. Blend in yogurt. Add whipping cream and blend until well combined. Pour into baking pan, cover and freeze until almost solid, about 1 hour.

2. Break up frozen strawberry mixture. Scrape a few chunks at a time into clean blender and purée on high speed.

3. Scrape into an airtight container, cover and freeze for at least 4 hours, until firm, or for up to 3 days. Soften at room temperature for 15 minutes before serving.

MAKES 4 TO
6 SERVINGS

This cheesecake-like mousse is smooth, rich and luxurious.

Strawberry Mousse

1	envelope (1/4 oz/7 g) powdered unflavored gelatin	1
2 tbsp	water	25 mL
1	package (8 oz/250 g) cream cheese, softened	1
1 cup	fresh or frozen strawberries	250 mL
1/2 cup	whipping (35%) cream	125 mL
1/2 cup	orange juice	125 mL
2 tbsp	granulated sugar	25 mL
1 tsp	vanilla	5 mL

1. In a small saucepan, sprinkle gelatin over water; let stand for 5 minutes. Melt over low heat for 2 to 3 minutes, or until gelatin is melted and clear.

2. Meanwhile, in blender, on high speed, purée cream cheese, strawberries, whipping cream, orange juice, sugar and vanilla until smooth. Add gelatin and purée.

3. Pour into custard cups, cover and refrigerate for at least 1 hour, until set, or for up to 3 days.

A simple and lovely winter dessert, you can chill the mousse in wine or cocktail glasses for a pretty presentation.

Citrus and Rum Mousse

● *Preheat broiler*
● *8- or 9-inch (2 or 2.5 L) baking dish, buttered*

2	oranges	2
1	grapefruit	1
1½ tsp	powdered unflavored gelatin	7 mL
1 tsp	butter	5 mL
¼ cup	packed dark brown sugar	50 mL
2 tbsp	dark rum	25 mL
1 cup	whipping (35%) cream	250 mL

1. Remove peel and pith from oranges and grapefruit. Over a bowl, cut out flesh between membranes, reserving juice and segments separately.

2. Pour juice into a small saucepan, sprinkle with gelatin and let stand for 5 minutes. Heat juice mixture over low heat, stirring, for 2 to 3 minutes, or until gelatin is melted and clear. Let cool.

3. Place orange and grapefruit segments in prepared pan. Sprinkle with sugar and rum. Broil until sugar is melted, about 5 minutes. Let cool.

4. In blender, on high speed, whip cream, scraping down sides as necessary, until thick. Add orange and grapefruit and any juices; blend on low speed until smooth. Add gelatin mixture and blend on low speed until thoroughly mixed.

5. Pour into a bowl or glasses and refrigerate for at least 4 hours, until set, or for up to 3 days.

*Parfaits are coming
back into fashion.
They look pretty and
are easy to make.*

Raspberry Mousse Parfaits

3½ cups	fresh raspberries, divided	875 mL
2 tbsp	granulated sugar	25 mL
1½ cups	whipping (35%) cream	375 mL
3 cups	cubed prepared pound cake or angel food cake	750 mL
⅓ cup	orange juice	75 mL

1. In blender, on high speed, purée 1 cup (250 mL) of the raspberries and sugar. Strain through a fine sieve into a bowl, pressing to remove seeds.

2. In same blender, whip cream, scraping down sides as necessary, until very thick. Add raspberry purée and pulse to blend.

3. In a medium bowl, toss cake cubes with orange juice and let stand for 1 minute until juice is absorbed.

4. Divide one-quarter of the soaked cake among 4 bowls or large wine glasses. Divide one-quarter of the remaining raspberries and place on top of cake, then top evenly with one-quarter of the cream mixture. Repeat layers three more times. Garnish with the remaining raspberries.

Rhubarb and Strawberry Jelly

1	strip (2 inches/5 cm long) orange zest	1
2 cups	chopped fresh or frozen rhubarb	500 mL
2 cups	sliced fresh strawberries	500 mL
1 cup	dry white wine	250 mL
2/3 cup	water	150 mL
1/2 cup	granulated sugar	125 mL
2 tbsp	powdered unflavored gelatin	25 mL
3 tbsp	cold water	45 mL

Garnish

1 cup	whipped cream	250 mL
1 cup	sliced fresh strawberries	250 mL

1. In a large saucepan, bring orange zest, rhubarb, strawberries, wine, the 2/3 cup (150 mL) water and sugar to a boil. Reduce heat and simmer, uncovered, until rhubarb is broken up, about 10 minutes. Let cool slightly.

2. In a small saucepan, sprinkle gelatin over cold water; let stand for 5 minutes. Heat over low heat for 2 to 3 minutes, or until gelatin is melted and clear.

3. Meanwhile, in blender, on high speed, purée rhubarb mixture. Strain through a fine sieve into gelatin mixture; discard solids. Stir to combine.

4. Divide among large wine goblets, cover loosely and refrigerate for about 6 hours, until set, or for up to 3 days.

5. Top each glass with whipped cream and strawberries.

This nutty, European-style torte can be garnished with fresh raspberries and shaved bittersweet chocolate, if desired.

Hazelnut Torte

- Preheat oven to 350°F (180°C)
- Rimmed baking sheet
- 9-inch (23 cm) springform pan, generously greased and bottom lined with parchment or waxed paper

1 cup	hazelnuts	250 mL
4	eggs	4
¾ cup	granulated sugar	175 mL
2 tbsp	all-purpose flour	25 mL
2½ tsp	baking powder	12 mL
1½ cups	whipping (35%) cream	375 mL
¼ cup	confectioner's (icing) sugar, sifted (approx.)	50 mL
1 tbsp	brandy (or 1 tsp/5 mL vanilla)	15 mL

1. On baking sheet, toast hazelnuts in preheated oven until fragrant and skins begin to loosen, about 10 minutes. Rub nuts in a folded tea towel to slough off skins; discard skins. Set nuts aside.

2. In blender, on high speed, blend eggs and sugar until very smooth and light. Add nuts and blend until very finely chopped. With motor running on low speed, through hole in top, add flour and baking powder. Blend until just combined.

3. Pour into prepared pan and bake until puffed and brown and a tester inserted in the center comes out clean, about 15 minutes. Let cool in pan for 5 minutes, then remove from pan and cool on a rack. Remove parchment paper.

4. In clean blender, on low speed, blend whipping cream, sugar and brandy until fluffy. Adjust sweetness as desired. Serve on the side with cake.

*The flavor of this
classic ricotta cake
with rum-soaked
raisins and citrus peel
is reminiscent of
baked rice pudding.*

Italian-Style Ricotta Cheesecake

● *9-inch (23 cm) springform pan*

2	containers (each 1 lb/454 g) extra-smooth ricotta cheese	2
½ cup	raisins	125 mL
3 tbsp	dark rum	45 mL
1	slice dry bread, torn into small pieces	1
1 tbsp	butter, softened	15 mL
5	eggs	5
¾ cup	granulated sugar	175 mL
Pinch	salt	Pinch
½ cup	whipping (35%) cream	125 mL
	Grated zest of 1 lemon	
	Grated zest of 1 orange	
½ cup	pine nuts	125 mL

1. Place ricotta in a cheesecloth-lined strainer set over a large bowl. Cover with plastic wrap and refrigerate for at least 8 hours or for up to 24 hours. Discard whey (or reserve for another use, such as baking bread); set ricotta aside.

2. In a small bowl, combine raisins and rum. Let stand, tossing occasionally, until most of the rum is absorbed, about 30 minutes. Preheat oven to 375°F (190°C).

3. Meanwhile, in blender, on low speed, chop bread to make about ¼ cup (50 mL) fine crumbs.

4. Spread bottom and sides of springform pan with butter. Coat pan with bread crumbs, shaking out any extra crumbs. Set aside.

5. In clean blender, on high speed, blend eggs, sugar and salt until thick and pale yellow. With motor running on low speed, through hole in top, add ricotta, 1 tbsp (15 mL) at a time, then add whipping cream, lemon zest and orange zest. Blend until smooth. Stir in raisins and any remaining rum.

6. Scrape into prepared pan and sprinkle with pine nuts. Bake in preheated oven until golden brown and set in center, about 1 hour. Let cool completely in pan on a rack. Remove from pan and transfer to a plate. Serve at room temperature or cover and refrigerate until chilled, about 4 hours.

MAKES 10 TO 12 SERVINGS

This standard has served many a busy household well. It takes minutes to put together and is a real crowd-pleaser. You can replace the almond cookies with vanilla wafers, graham crackers or other cookies to taste.

TIP

To make cookie crumbs, break cookies into small pieces and pulse 1 cup (250 mL) at a time in blender.

No-Bake Lemon Cheesecake

● *9-inch (23 cm) pie plate or springform pan*

2 cups	crushed almond cookies	500 mL
½ cup	butter, melted	125 mL
1	package (8 oz/250 g) cream cheese, softened	1
1	can (10 oz/300 mL) sweetened condensed milk	1
1 tsp	grated lemon zest	5 mL
½ cup	freshly squeezed lemon juice	125 mL
¼ tsp	vanilla	1 mL

1. In a bowl, mix cookie crumbs and butter until well combined. Press into pie plate.

2. In blender, on low speed, blend cream cheese, condensed milk, lemon zest, lemon juice and vanilla until smooth. Pour into shell. Cover and refrigerate for at least 4 hours, until firm, or for up to 3 days.

Using the blender is a great way to cut down on the mess of preparing this impressive dessert.

TIPS

To make graham wafer crumbs, break graham wafers into small pieces and pulse ¾ cup (175 mL) at a time in blender.

Melt chocolate in a heatproof bowl over hot, but not boiling, water.

White Chocolate Cheesecake

● *Preheat oven to 350°F (180°C)*
● *9-inch (23 cm) springform pan*

Crust

½ cup	whole blanched almonds	125 mL
3 tbsp	granulated sugar	45 mL
1½ cups	graham wafer crumbs (about 20 wafers)	375 mL
⅓ cup	melted butter	75 mL

Cheesecake

3	eggs	3
6 oz	white chocolate, melted (see tip, at left) and slightly cooled	175 g
1 cup	sour cream	250 mL
¾ cup	granulated sugar	175 mL
½ tsp	vanilla	2 mL
2	packages (each 8 oz/250g) cream cheese, softened	2
1	package (10 oz/300 g) frozen unsweetened raspberries, thawed and drained	1

1. *Prepare the crust:* In blender, on high speed, blend almonds and sugar until finely chopped. Pulse in graham wafer crumbs and butter until combined. Press into pan and bake in preheated oven until brown and firm, about 10 minutes. Set aside.

2. *Prepare the cheesecake:* In clean blender, on high speed, blend eggs, chocolate, sour cream, sugar and vanilla until smooth. With motor running, through hole in top, add cream cheese, about 1 tbsp (15 mL) at a time. Blend until smooth. Pour 4 cups (1 L) of cheese mixture over crust.

3. Add raspberries to remaining mixture in blender and blend on high speed until smooth. Strain through a fine sieve into a bowl, pressing to remove seeds.

4. Drop five circles of raspberry mixture around edges of cheese mixture; drop one circle in center. With the tip of a knife, swirl each raspberry circle slightly into cheese mixture to create a marbled effect.

5. Bake at 350°F (180°C) until almost set, about 45 minutes. Let cool completely in pan on a rack. Remove from pan and transfer to a plate. Cover and refrigerate for at least 4 hours, until chilled, or for up to 3 days.

Apple Fritters

This batter is also terrific with bananas, pears and thinly sliced pumpkin. Serve with Butter Pecan Ice Cream (see recipe, page 186) for a real Southern treat.

TIP

Sprinkle with confectioner's (icing) sugar for an attractive presentation.

● *Deep skillet or deep-fryer, filled with at least 2 inches (5 cm) vegetable oil*
● *Preheat vegetable oil to 375°F (190°C)*

1	egg	1
1 cup	unsweetened apple juice	250 mL
1 cup	all-purpose flour	250 mL
2 tbsp	granulated sugar	25 mL
1 $\frac{1}{2}$ tsp	baking powder	7 mL
$\frac{1}{2}$ tsp	salt	2 mL
$\frac{1}{2}$ tsp	ground cinnamon	2 mL
$\frac{1}{4}$ tsp	ground nutmeg	1 mL
4	large cooking apples	4

1. In blender, on high speed, purée egg and apple juice.

2. In a small bowl, whisk together flour, sugar, baking powder, salt, cinnamon and nutmeg.

3. With motor running on low speed, through hole in top, gradually add flour mixture to blender until smooth. Transfer to a bowl and let stand for 20 minutes.

4. Meanwhile, peel, core and slice apples into $\frac{1}{2}$-inch (1 cm) thick rings. Dip apple rings in batter a few at a time and fry in hot oil, turning once, for 3 to 4 minutes, or until golden brown. Drain on paper towels. Repeat with remaining apples and batter.

*You may not think to
make a pumpkin-style
pie with another
squash, but butternut
has a wonderful
caramel flavor that is
well suited to desserts.*

Butternut Squash Pie

● *9-inch (23 cm) pie plate*

4 lbs	butternut squash, cut into large chunks	2 kg
¼ cup	walnut halves	50 mL
1 ¼ cups	all-purpose flour	300 mL
½ tsp	salt	2 mL
⅓ cup	butter, shortening or lard	75 mL
¼ cup	ice water	50 mL
1 ⅓ cups	evaporated milk	325 mL
½ cup	granulated sugar	125 mL
¼ cup	packed brown sugar	50 mL
1 tsp	ground cinnamon	5 mL
½ tsp	ground ginger	2 mL
½ tsp	ground nutmeg	2 mL
3	eggs	3
	Whipped cream	

1. Arrange squash in a steamer basket fitted over a saucepan of boiling water. Cover and steam until very soft, about 20 minutes. Scoop out flesh to measure 4 cups (1 L). Scrape into a skillet and cook over medium heat, stirring and scraping up bottom, until reduced by half and darkened to deep orange, about 10 minutes. Let cool.

2. Meanwhile, in blender, pulse walnuts until finely chopped. Add flour and salt; blend on low speed until well combined. With motor running on low speed, through hole in top, add butter until just combined, with a few large pieces still remaining. Pulse in ice water until pastry clumps.

3. On a floured surface, roll out dough to a 12-inch (30 cm) diameter circle. Transfer to pie plate and trim edges to $\frac{1}{2}$ inch (1 cm) beyond rim; fold under extra pastry and flute edges as desired. Cover and refrigerate until ready to use or for up to 1 day. Meanwhile, preheat oven to 375°F (190°C).

4. In clean blender, on high speed, blend caramelized squash, evaporated milk, sugar, brown sugar, cinnamon, ginger and nutmeg until smooth. Pulse in eggs, one at a time, until well combined.

5. Pour into pie crust and cover edges with foil. Bake for 25 minutes, then remove foil. Bake until a knife inserted in the center comes out clean, about 20 minutes. Let cool completely in pan on a rack. Top with whipped cream.

Because of the Jewish prohibition against mixing meat and milk, there are many dairy restaurants that serve only dairy dishes and fish. Anybody who has ever been to a Jewish dairy restaurant has enjoyed wonderful cheese blintzes. They are easy to make and make a nice lunch or supper, or dessert after a light dinner.

TIPS

To make cinnamon sugar, combine 2 tbsp (25 mL) granulated sugar with $\frac{1}{2}$ tsp (2 mL) ground cinnamon.

Dry cottage cheese and farmer's cheese are the same thing.

Sweet Cheese Blintzes

● *6-inch (15 cm) crêpe pan or nonstick skillet*

Batter

3	eggs	3
1 $\frac{1}{2}$ cups	milk	375 mL
3 tbsp	melted butter or vegetable oil	45 mL
1 tbsp	granulated sugar	15 mL
1 tsp	salt	5 mL
1 cup	all-purpose flour	250 mL
1 tbsp	vegetable oil (approx.)	15 mL

Filling

1	egg	1
1 cup	dry cottage cheese	250 mL
$\frac{1}{2}$ cup	sour cream	125 mL
$\frac{1}{2}$ cup	cream cheese, softened	125 mL
1 tbsp	liquid honey (or 2 tsp/10 mL granulated sugar)	15 mL
$\frac{1}{2}$ tsp	ground cinnamon	2 mL
Generous pinch	ground nutmeg	Generous pinch
Generous pinch	freshly ground white pepper	Generous pinch
2 tbsp	butter	25 mL
2 tbsp	cinnamon sugar (optional, see tip at left)	25 mL

1. *Prepare the batter:* In blender, on low speed, blend eggs, milk, butter, sugar and salt until combined. With motor running on high speed, through hole in top, add flour. Blend until smooth, scraping down sides once or twice. Let stand for 1 hour.

2. Heat crêpe pan over medium-high heat. Brush lightly with oil. Pour $\frac{1}{4}$ cup (50 mL) batter into pan and swirl to coat. Cook until bottom is lightly browned, about 1 minute; flip and lightly brown the other side. Remove to a plate and cover with waxed paper. Repeat with remaining batter. Let cool.

3. *Prepare the filling:* In clean blender, on high speed, blend egg, cottage cheese, sour cream, cream cheese, honey, cinnamon, nutmeg and white pepper until smooth.

4. Spoon a generous 1 tbsp (15 mL) filling into the center of each crêpe. Fold over top and bottom, then sides, to make a sealed envelope.

5. In a large skillet, melt butter over medium heat. Cook blintzes in batches, turning once, until browned on both sides and filling is hot, about 3 minutes. Sprinkle with cinnamon sugar, if desired.

Fruit purée is a great lower-fat substitute for butter in these moist, tasty muffins. The secret to its tenderness? Don't over-mix the batter; pulse it until just smooth.

Piña Colada Muffins

● *Preheat oven to 400°F (200°C)*
● *12-cup muffin pan, greased or lined with paper liners*

¾ cup	shredded coconut, divided	175 mL
1 cup	all-purpose flour	250 mL
½ cup	whole wheat flour	125 mL
1 tbsp	baking powder	15 mL
½ tsp	baking soda	2 mL
½ tsp	salt	2 mL
1	can (14 oz/398 mL) crushed pineapple, drained	1
1	egg	1
½ cup	granulated sugar	125 mL
½ cup	light sour cream	125 mL
¼ cup	vegetable oil	50 mL
1 tsp	vanilla	5 mL

1. Set aside ⅓ cup (75 mL) of the coconut. In a medium bowl, whisk together the remaining coconut, flour, whole wheat flour, baking powder, baking soda and salt. Set aside.

2. In blender, on high speed, purée pineapple. Add egg, sugar, sour cream, vegetable oil and vanilla; blend until smooth. Add flour mixture and pulse until just combined.

3. Divide batter among muffin cups and sprinkle tops with reserved coconut. Bake in preheated oven until golden and a tester inserted in the center comes out clean, about 20 minutes. Let cool in pan on a rack for 5 minutes. Remove from pan and let cool completely on rack.

Moist and irresistable,
these individual carrot
cakes will delight
your family.

Carrot Cake Muffins

● *Preheat oven to 400°F (200°C)*
● *12-cup muffin pan, greased or lined with paper liners*

1 cup	all-purpose flour	250 mL
½ cup	whole wheat flour	125 mL
1 tbsp	baking powder	15 mL
1 tsp	ground cinnamon	5 mL
½ tsp	baking soda	2 mL
½ tsp	salt	2 mL
¼ tsp	ground cloves	1 mL
1¾ cup	cooked chopped carrots or 1 can (14 oz/398 mL) carrots, drained	425 mL
1	egg	1
½ cup	light sour cream	125 mL
¼ cup	granulated sugar	50 mL
¼ cup	packed brown sugar	50 mL
¼ cup	vegetable oil	50 mL
1 tsp	vanilla	5 mL

1. In a small bowl, whisk together all-purpose flour, whole wheat flour, baking powder, cinnamon, baking soda, salt and cloves. Set aside.

2. In blender, on high speed, purée carrots. Add egg, sour cream, sugar, brown sugar, vegetable oil and vanilla; blend until smooth. Add flour mixture and pulse until just combined.

3. Divide batter among muffin cups and bake in preheated oven until a tester inserted in the center comes out clean, about 20 minutes. Let cool in pan on a rack for 5 minutes. Remove from pan and let cool completely on rack.

This is a thicker, more sweet-and-sour version of applesauce.

Apple Butter

2 lbs	red-skinned cooking apples, such as Northern Spy or Gravenstein (about 6)	1 kg
1 cup	water	250 mL
1/3 cup	cider vinegar	75 mL
1 cup	granulated sugar	250 mL
2 tsp	grated lemon zest	10 mL
2 tbsp	freshly squeezed lemon juice	25 mL
1 tsp	ground cinnamon	5 mL
1/4 tsp	ground nutmeg	1 mL
1/4 tsp	ground allspice	1 mL
Pinch	salt	Pinch

1. Core and cut apples into quarters, without peeling. In a large saucepan, bring apples, water and vinegar to a boil. Cover, reduce heat to low and simmer gently until apples are very soft, about 20 minutes. Remove from heat and let cool for 5 minutes.

2. Transfer to blender, in batches, and purée on high speed. Strain through a sieve, forcing pulp into a large bowl.

3. Place pulp and sugar in a clean saucepan over medium heat and stir to dissolve sugar. Add lemon zest, lemon juice, cinnamon, nutmeg, allspice and salt. Taste and adjust seasonings if necessary. Reduce heat to low and simmer until very thick and smooth, about 45 minutes. Let cool.

4. *Make ahead:* Pour into sealable decorative jars. Seal and refrigerate for up to 2 weeks or freeze for up to 2 months.

Fruit Syrup

*This syrup is great
on top of pancakes,
waffles or ice cream.*

1 cup	granulated sugar	250 mL
½ cup	water	125 mL
2 cups	strawberries, blueberries, raspberries or blackberries, or chopped peeled fruit, such as apples, pears, peaches, mangoes or apricots	500 mL
1 tbsp	freshly squeezed lemon juice	15 mL
½ tsp	vanilla	2 mL

1. In a large saucepan, bring sugar and water to a boil, stirring until sugar is dissolved. Boil for 5 minutes. Add fruit, lemon juice and vanilla. Reduce heat and simmer, uncovered, until fruit is tender, about 5 minutes. Let cool.

2. Transfer to blender and purée on high speed. Strain through a fine sieve, pressing to remove seeds.

3. *Make ahead:* Pour into sealable decorative jars. Seal and refrigerate for up to 1 week.

Lemon Sauce

**MAKES ABOUT
1¼ CUPS (300 ML)**

*This tart sauce is
wonderful on plain
cake, such as pound
cake, or on puddings.*

1	lemon	1
1 cup	water	250 mL
¼ cup	butter, softened	50 mL
3 tbsp	granulated sugar	45 mL
2 tbsp	cornstarch	25 mL

1. With a vegetable peeler, peel zest of lemon and cut off white pith. Cut lemon in half, seed and chop. Place lemon zest and flesh in blender and add water, butter, sugar and cornstarch; purée on high speed.

2. Strain through a fine sieve into a small saucepan. Bring to a boil over medium heat, stirring. Reduce heat and simmer, stirring often, until syrupy, about 5 minutes. Let cool.

3. *Make ahead:* Pour into sealable decorative jars. Seal and refrigerate for up to 2 weeks. Bring to room temperature before serving.

This sweet fruity sauce is fantastic warm or cold over ice cream, crêpes, sponge cake and whipped cream or custard. Use any fruit juice, such as raspberry juice cocktail or orange juice.

Strawberry-Vodka Sauce

2 cups	fresh or frozen strawberries	500 mL
1/3 cup	granulated sugar	75 mL
1/4 cup	fruit juice	50 mL
2 tbsp	freshly squeezed lemon juice	25 mL
1/4 cup	vodka	50 mL
1 tsp	vanilla	5 mL

1. In a medium saucepan, bring strawberries, sugar, fruit juice and lemon juice to a boil. Reduce heat and simmer until thickened, about 5 minutes. Stir in vodka and vanilla. Let cool slightly.

2. Transfer to blender and purée on high speed.

3. *Make ahead:* Pour into sealable decorative jars. Seal and refrigerate for up to 5 days. Warm before serving, if desired.

This decadent sauce is wonderful warm or cold over ice cream or fresh fruit salad.

Peach Sauce

3/4 cup	granulated sugar	175 mL
3/4 cup	water	175 mL
1 1/2 cups	sliced fresh or frozen peaches	375 mL
1/3 cup	whipping (35%) cream	75 mL
4 tsp	freshly squeezed lemon juice	20 mL
1/2 tsp	vanilla	2 mL

1. In a deep saucepan, over medium heat, stir sugar and water until sugar is dissolved. Bring to a boil. Boil, without stirring, until amber-colored. Remove from heat. Averting face, add peaches and whipping cream. Return to heat and simmer, stirring, until thickened, about 3 minutes. Let cool slightly.

2. Transfer to blender and add lemon juice and vanilla; blend on high speed until smooth.

3. *Make ahead:* Refrigerate for up to 1 week. Warm before serving.

This is a convenient last-minute sauce for topping ice cream, cakes or other desserts.

TIP

After the chocolate is melted, you can flavor this sauce with 2 tsp (10 mL) brandy, rum or fruit eau-de-vie or liqueur.

Chocolate Sauce

2 oz	semi-sweet chocolate	60 g
1 oz	milk chocolate	30 g
¼ tsp	vanilla	1 mL
⅓ cup	whipping (35%) cream	75 mL
1 tbsp	butter	15 mL

1. In blender, on low speed, blend semi-sweet chocolate, milk chocolate and vanilla until finely chopped.

2. In a small saucepan, over medium-high heat, heat whipping cream and butter until bubbling at the edges.

3. With blender motor running at low speed, through hole in top, pour in cream mixture. Blend until chocolate is thoroughly melted. Serve warm.

4. *Make ahead:* Pour into sealable decorative jars. Seal and refrigerate for up to 1 week. Warm before serving.

Thick Chocolate Sauce

6 oz	bittersweet chocolate, coarsely chopped	175 g
1 cup	whipping (35%) cream	250 mL
2 tbsp	corn syrup	25 mL
⅓ cup	sour cream	75 mL

1. In blender, pulse chocolate until finely chopped.

2. In a small saucepan, bring whipping cream and corn syrup to a boil. Remove from heat. (Or, in a small microwave-safe bowl, microwave whipping cream and corn syrup on High for 1 to 2 minutes, or until boiling.)

3. Transfer to blender with chocolate and pulse until smooth and thick. Add sour cream and blend on high speed until smooth. Let stand until thickened, about 15 minutes.

4. *Make-ahead:* Pour into sealable decorative jars. Seal and refrigerate for up to 1 week. Warm before serving.

Velvety and delicious, this sauce is great over any fresh fruit, but is particularly nice with tropical fruit.

TIP

Toast coconut on a baking sheet in a 375°F (190°C) oven or in a dry skillet over medium heat, stirring often.

White Chocolate Coconut Sauce

⅓ cup	whipping (35%) cream	75 mL
4 oz	good-quality white chocolate	125 g
¼ cup	shredded sweetened coconut, toasted (see tip, at left)	50 mL
¼ cup	coconut milk	50 mL
Dash	coconut extract	Dash

1. In a small saucepan, bring whipping cream to a boil.

2. In blender, pulse chocolate and coconut until finely chopped. Pour in hot cream and pulse until smooth.

3. Scrape into a bowl and let cool to room temperature. Stir in coconut milk and coconut extract.

4. *Make ahead:* Pour into sealable decorative jars. Seal and refrigerate for up to 3 days. Bring to room temperature before serving.

MAKES ABOUT 1½ CUPS (375 ML) OR 6 TO 8 SERVINGS

This dip is best served with seasonal fresh fruit, either as an informal summer dessert or as the centerpiece to a party fruit tray.

TIP

Flavor with 1 tsp (5 mL) hazelnut liqueur, Kirsch or orange liqueur, if desired.

Chocolate Cheesecake Dip

3 oz	bittersweet chocolate, melted	90 g
⅓ cup	half-and-half (10%) cream	75 mL
2 tbsp	granulated sugar	25 mL
½ tsp	vanilla	2 mL
1	package (8 oz/250 g) cream cheese, cut into cubes, softened	1
	Assorted fruit (such as grapes, melon, pineapple and strawberries)	

1. In blender, on high speed, blend chocolate, cream, sugar and vanilla until combined. With motor running, through hole in top, add cream cheese cubes, one at a time. Blend until smooth.

2. Scrape into a serving bowl and serve with fresh fruit.

Smoothies and Other Drinks

This vegetable smoothie is fresh and pungent.

Gazpacho Smoothie

2	fresh tomatoes, peeled	2
1	small clove garlic, smashed	1
1 cup	chopped peeled and seeded cucumber	250 mL
1 cup	tomato juice	250 mL
2 tsp	freshly squeezed lemon juice	10 mL
Pinch	salt	Pinch
Pinch	freshly ground black pepper	Pinch
6	ice cubes	6

1. In blender, on high speed, purée tomatoes, garlic, cucumber, tomato juice, lemon juice, salt, pepper and ice.

This is much fresher, thicker and more delicious than canned vegetable cocktail.

Fresh Vegetable Smoothie

2	tomatoes, peeled	2
1	medium peeled cooked or canned beet	1
1 cup	tomato juice or tomato-clam juice	250 mL
1/2 cup	carrot juice	125 mL
Pinch	salt	Pinch
Pinch	freshly ground black pepper	Pinch
6	ice cubes	6
2	stalks celery	2

1. In blender, on high speed, purée tomatoes, beet, tomato juice, carrot juice, salt, pepper and ice, about 3 minutes. Pour into tall glasses and garnish with celery stalks.

This vibrant smoothie is loaded with nutrients and has a rich creaminess from the avocado.

Green Smoothie

9	ice cubes	9
1	avocado, peeled, pitted and chopped	1
1	small clove garlic, smashed	1
2 cups	chopped seeded cucumber (unpeeled)	500 mL
1 cup	packed spinach leaves	250 mL
2/3 cup	water	150 mL
2 tbsp	freshly squeezed lemon juice or lime juice	25 mL
1 tbsp	fresh dill	15 mL
1/4 tsp	salt	1 mL
1/4 tsp	freshly ground black pepper	1 mL

1. In blender, on low speed, chop ice. Add avocado, garlic, cucumber, spinach, water, lemon juice, dill, salt and pepper; purée on high speed, about 3 minutes.

In Asia and the Middle East, refreshing yogurt-based drinks are very popular and come in all sorts of sweet and savory flavors. This cucumber drink is great on a hot summer day. Garnish with mint leaves, if desired.

Cucumber Yogurt Smoothie

2 cups	chopped peeled and seeded cucumber	500 mL
1 cup	sparkling water	250 mL
1/2 cup	plain yogurt	125 mL
1/4 cup	lightly packed fresh mint leaves	50 mL
6	ice cubes	6

1. In blender, on high speed, purée cucumber, sparkling water, yogurt, mint and ice.

Fruit and Veggies Smoothie

1 cup	frozen blueberries	250 mL
¾ cup	carrot-orange cocktail	175 mL
¾ cup	cranberry cocktail	175 mL
⅓ cup	silken tofu	75 mL
2 tbsp	orange juice concentrate, thawed	25 mL
1 tbsp	wheat bran	15 mL
1 tbsp	ground flaxseed	15 mL
1 tsp	liquid honey	5 mL

1. In blender, on high speed, purée blueberries, carrot-orange cocktail, cranberry cocktail, tofu, orange juice concentrate, bran, flaxseed and honey.

Mulled Apple Smoothie

2	apples, peeled, cored and chopped	2
½	banana	½
1 cup	unsweetened apple cider	250 mL
2 tsp	packed dark brown sugar	10 mL
¼ tsp	ground cinnamon	1 mL
Pinch	ground nutmeg	Pinch

1. In blender, on high speed, purée apples, banana, apple cider, sugar, cinnamon and nutmeg.

Adding ice will chill this sweet fruit smoothie and make it a bit slushier.

Apple Apricot Smoothie

4	fresh or canned, drained pitted apricots	4
1	apple, peeled, cored and chopped	1
1	banana	1
1 cup	unsweetened apple cider or juice	250 mL
¾ cup	vanilla-flavored yogurt	175 mL
1 tbsp	liquid honey	15 mL
6	ice cubes (optional)	6

1. In blender, on high speed, purée apricots, apple, banana, apple cider, yogurt, honey and ice (if using).

This simple smoothie is a great way to get picky eaters to start eating breakfast.

TIP

If you prefer, you can replace the strawberries with raspberries.

Pink Berry Smoothie

½	banana	½
1 cup	vanilla-flavored yogurt	250 mL
¾ cup	milk	175 mL
¾ cup	fruit punch or berry cocktail	175 mL
½ cup	fresh or frozen strawberries	125 mL
1 tsp	liquid honey	5 mL

1. In blender, on high speed, purée banana, yogurt, milk, fruit punch, strawberries and honey.

The banana gives a rich smoothness to this lower-fat smoothie.

Blueberry Smoothie

½	banana	½
1 cup	fresh or frozen blueberries	250 mL
¾ cup	skim milk	175 mL
¼ cup	nonfat vanilla-flavored yogurt	50 mL
¼ tsp	ground cinnamon	1 mL
4	ice cubes	4

1. In blender, on high speed, purée banana, blueberries, milk, yogurt, cinnamon and ice.

Sour Cherry Smoothie

2 cups	fresh or frozen strawberries or raspberries	500 mL
1 cup	pitted sour cherries	250 mL
1/2 cup	water	125 mL
1 tbsp	almond butter	15 mL
2 tsp	liquid honey	10 mL
1/4 tsp	almond extract	1 mL

1. In blender, on high speed, purée strawberries, cherries, water, almond butter, honey and almond extract.

Coconut Lime Smoothie

MAKES 2 SERVINGS

This smoothie is packed with tropical flavor.

TIP

You can replace the mango with papaya or pineapple.

1/2	banana	1/2
1 cup	chopped peeled mango	250 mL
1 cup	milk	250 mL
1/4 cup	coconut milk	50 mL
2 tsp	finely grated lime zest	10 mL
1 tbsp	freshly squeezed lime juice	15 mL
1 tsp	packed brown sugar	5 mL

1. In blender, on high speed, purée banana, mango, milk, coconut milk, lime zest, lime juice and brown sugar.

Ruby Red Smoothie

MAKES 2 SERVINGS

This smoothie has a gorgeous pink color and, as a change from a glass of juice or half a grapefruit, is a creative way to get a serving of citrus fruit in the morning.

1	ruby red grapefruit	1
1	banana	1
1 cup	milk, plain yogurt or buttermilk	250 mL
2 tbsp	orange juice concentrate, thawed	25 mL

1. Cut off peel and white pith from grapefruit; cut into quarters and remove any seeds.
2. In blender, on high speed, purée grapefruit, banana, milk and orange juice concentrate, about 3 minutes.

A great start to the morning, this smoothie is redolent of hot summer days.

TIP

To peel the peach, submerge it in boiling water for 10 to 15 seconds to loosen the skin.

Summer Smoothie

2 tbsp	wheat germ	25 mL
2	peaches, peeled and pitted	2
2 cups	buttermilk	500 mL
1 cup	wild or cultivated blueberries	250 mL
2 tsp	liquid honey	10 mL

1. In a dry heavy-bottomed skillet wiped clean of any lingering oil, over medium heat, toast wheat germ, shaking pan, for 4 to 6 minutes, or until fragrant.

2. Transfer to blender and add peach, buttermilk, blueberries and honey; purée on high speed.

MAKES 2 SERVINGS

This gingery shake, loaded with vitamin A from the mango and potassium from the banana, is a great start to the day.

Mango Ginger Smoothie

1	mango, peeled and chopped	1
½	banana	½
1 cup	mango nectar or orange juice	250 mL
½ cup	plain yogurt	125 mL
2 tsp	granulated sugar or liquid honey	10 mL
1 tsp	finely grated gingerroot	5 mL

1. In blender, on high speed, purée mango, banana, mango nectar, yogurt, sugar and ginger.

Mango Green Tea Custard Smoothie

3	bags green tea (or 1 tbsp (15 mL) loose tea)	3
1 cup	half-and-half (10%) cream	250 mL
2 tbsp	granulated sugar, divided	25 mL
3	egg yolks	3
½ tsp	vanilla	2 mL
2	mangoes	2
½ cup	milk	125 mL

1. In small saucepan, over medium heat, heat tea bags, cream and 1 tbsp (15 mL) of the sugar until steaming, bubbles form around the edge and tea is fragrant, about 3 minutes.

2. Meanwhile, in a small bowl, whisk egg yolks with the remaining 1 tbsp (15 mL) sugar. In a thin stream, whisk hot tea mixture into yolk mixture. Stir back into pan and cook, stirring constantly, until thick enough to coat the spoon, about 5 minutes.

3. Strain into a clean bowl and stir in vanilla. Place plastic wrap directly on surface of custard and let cool. Refrigerate for at least 1 hour, until cold, or for up to 3 days.

4. Peel, pit and chop mangoes. Scrape chilled custard into blender and add mangoes and milk; purée on high speed.

Neapolitan Smoothie

1 cup	chocolate milk	250 mL
1 cup	frozen strawberries	250 mL
1 cup	vanilla-flavored yogurt	250 mL
¼ cup	skim milk powder	50 mL

1. In blender, on high speed, purée chocolate milk, strawberries, yogurt and milk powder.

Rhubarb Smoothie

2 cups	chopped fresh or frozen rhubarb	500 mL
1/2 cup	water	125 mL
1/4 cup	liquid honey	50 mL
1 tsp	vanilla	5 mL
1 cup	orange juice	250 mL
6	ice cubes	6

1. In a medium saucepan, bring rhubarb, water and honey to a boil. Cover, reduce heat to low and simmer until tender and falling apart, about 10 minutes. Stir in vanilla. Let cool and refrigerate until cold.

2. Transfer to blender, add orange juice and ice cubes; purée on high speed.

Corn Smoothie

2 cups	cooked corn kernels or frozen corn, thawed	500 mL
2 cup	buttermilk	500 mL
1/4 tsp	granulated sugar	1 mL
1/4 tsp	salt	1 mL
Pinch	cayenne pepper (optional) Pinch	

1. In blender, on high speed, purée corn, buttermilk, sugar, salt and cayenne, if using.

Two Melon Shake

3 cups	coarsely chopped seeded bitter melon	750 mL
2 cups	cubed seedless watermelon	500 mL
6	ice cubes	6
Pinch	salt	Pinch

1. In blender, on high speed, purée bitter melon, watermelon, ice and salt.

Bitter Melon Shake

Bitter but absolutely refreshing, this shake is a wonderful summer pick-me-up.

3 cups	coarsely chopped seeded bitter melon	750 mL
8	ice cubes	8
1/4 tsp	salt	1 mL

1. In blender, on high speed, purée bitter melon, ice and salt.

Currant Shake

Serve as a simple summer dessert with vanilla wafers or as a snack. For a less sweet shake, halve the sugar.

1 cup	buttermilk	250 mL
1/2 cup	red currants (or 2/3 cup/150 mL black currants)	125 mL
1/2 cup	vanilla ice cream	125 mL
1/4 cup	granulated sugar or liquid honey	50 mL
	Fresh mint leaves	

1. In blender, on high speed, purée buttermilk, currants, ice cream and sugar. Pour into tall glasses and garnish with a few mint leaves, if desired.

Star Fruit Shake

The combination of cooling star fruit (carambola) and salt makes for an amazing summer drink, especially after exercising, when salt is needed.

3	star fruits	3
1 1/2 to 2 tbsp	granulated sugar or liquid honey	22 to 25 mL
1/2 tsp	sea salt	2 mL
	Juice of 2 limes	
8	ice cubes	8

1. Trim each rib of star fruits of waxy edges. Cut off each rib, discarding core and seeds.
2. In blender, on high speed, purée star fruit, sugar to taste, salt, lime juice and ice.

This tea and condensed milk drink is often served as bubble tea, with the addition of large, cooked tapioca pearls.

Green Tea "Milkshake"

2 tsp	green tea powder	10 mL
½ cup	boiling water	125 mL
3 tbsp	sweetened condensed milk (or to taste)	45 mL
16	ice cubes	16

1. In a small bowl, mix together green tea powder and water to form a paste.
2. Scrape into blender and add condensed milk and ice cubes; blend on high speed until smooth and slushy.

A sweet and fruity dairy-free shake.

Mango-Peach Soy Shake

1 cup	fresh or frozen chopped peaches	250 mL
½ cup	water	125 mL
⅔ cup	mango sorbet	150 mL
½ cup	silken or soft tofu	125 mL

1. In blender, on high speed, purée peaches and water. Add sorbet and tofu; blend until smooth and creamy.

In season, use fresh berries and add three ice cubes to maintain the texture. Strain out the seeds if you don't like the crunch.

Banana-Berry Rice Milkshake

2	bananas	2
2 cups	frozen mixed berries	500 mL
2 cups	vanilla-flavored rice milk	500 mL

1. In blender, on high speed, purée banana, berries and rice milk until smooth and creamy.

The combination of banana, ice and rice milk creates the body and texture of a real milkshake but with much less fat.

Banana Malted Rice Milkshake

1	banana	1
1 cup	vanilla-flavored rice milk, divided	250 mL
2 tbsp	malt powder (such as Ovaltine, Horlicks or Milo)	25 mL
3	ice cubes	3

1. In blender, on high speed, blend banana, $\frac{1}{2}$ cup (125 mL) of the rice milk and malt powder until smooth and no large chunks remain. Add the remaining $\frac{1}{2}$ cup (125 mL) rice milk and ice cubes; blend until smooth and creamy.

Variation

Chocolate-Banana Malted Rice Milkshake: Substitute chocolate-flavored rice milk for the vanilla rice milk.

Blend the fruit first to ensure that this shake is smooth and creamy.

Creamy Cantaloupe Rice Milkshake

1 $\frac{1}{2}$ cups	chopped very ripe cantaloupe	375 mL
3 tbsp	frozen orange juice concentrate	45 mL
$\frac{1}{2}$ cup	rice milk (vanilla-flavored or plain)	125 mL
6	ice cubes	6

1. In blender, on high speed, blend cantaloupe and orange juice concentrate until no large chunks remain. Add rice milk and ice cubes; blend until smooth and creamy.

Variation

Creamy Honeydew Rice Milkshake: Substitute honeydew melon for the cantaloupe and apple juice concentrate for the orange juice concentrate.

Vietnamese Milkshake

9	ice cubes	9
1/2	large mango, peeled, pitted and chopped	1/2
1/2	avocado, peeled, pitted and chopped	1/2
1/4 cup	water	50 mL
2 tbsp	sweetened condensed milk	25 mL
	Granulated sugar (optional)	

1. In blender, on low speed, chop ice. Add mango, avocado, water and condensed milk; purée on high speed. Pour into tall glasses and stir in sugar, if using.

Variation

Replace avocado with half of a small papaya or 3/4 cup (175 mL) drained canned papaya.

Creamy Coffee Slushy

1 1/2 cups	hot strong brewed coffee	375 mL
1/4 cup	granulated sugar	50 mL
1/3 cup	whipping (35%) cream	75 mL
1/3 cup	cold water	75 mL

1. In a measuring cup with a spout, stir coffee and sugar until sugar is dissolved. Pour into an ice cube tray and freeze until firm, about 4 hours.
2. Transfer cubes to blender and add whipping cream and water; purée on high speed until very thick.

Carrot-Pineapple Slushy

1 cup	grated peeled carrot	250 mL
1 cup	crushed pineapple, with juice	250 mL
1 cup	water	250 mL
6	ice cubes	6

1. In blender, on high speed, blend carrots, pineapple, water and ice cubes until smooth and slushy. Pour into chilled glasses or keep refrigerated until ready to serve.

Chai Slushy

2	oranges	2
2 cups	water	500 mL
6	star anise (or 1 tsp/5 mL anise seeds)	6
6	cardamom pods, crushed	6
2 tbsp	black tea leaves	25 mL
3 tbsp	sweetened condensed milk (or to taste)	45 mL
1 tsp	vanilla	5 mL
6	ice cubes	6

1. Remove peel from orange with a vegetable peeler, avoiding white pith; reserve flesh for another use.

2. In a small saucepan, bring water, orange peel, star anise and cardamom to a boil. Add tea. Remove from heat and let stand, covered, until cooled to room temperature, about 20 minutes.

3. Strain through a sieve into blender. Add condensed milk, vanilla and ice; blend on high speed until slushy. Pour into tall glasses.

Variation

Replace the sweetened condensed milk with 6 tbsp (90 mL) half-and-half (10%) cream and 2 tbsp (25 mL) granulated sugar.

This smoothie is cool and refreshing.

Lime Frost

9	ice cubes	9
1	banana	1
1 cup	vanilla-flavored yogurt	250 mL
3 tbsp	granulated sugar	45 mL
2 tsp	finely grated lime zest	10 mL
2 tbsp	freshly squeezed lime juice	25 mL
2	thin lime slices	2

1. In blender, on low speed, chop ice. Add banana, yogurt, sugar, lime zest and lime juice; purée on high speed. Pour into tall glasses and float a slice of lime on each.

This vibrant smoothie sparkles on your tongue.

Grape Blueberry Fizz

1 ½ cups	fresh or frozen blueberries	375 mL
1 cup	Concord grape juice	250 mL
½ cup	vanilla-flavored yogurt	125 mL
1 cup	sparkling water	250 mL

1. In blender, on high speed, purée blueberries, grape juice and yogurt. Pour in sparkling water and pulse to blend.

A few berries add a splash of red to this golden, creamy-tasting smoothie.

Nectarine Dream

2	nectarines or peaches, peeled, pitted and chopped	2
½	very ripe banana	½
1 cup	milk	250 mL
½ cup	fresh or frozen strawberries	125 mL
3 tbsp	sweetened condensed milk	45 mL

1. In blender, on high speed, purée nectarines, banana, milk, strawberries and condensed milk

Blueberry Lemonade

¼ cup	granulated sugar	50 mL
¼ cup	water	50 mL
1	strip (1 inch/2.5 cm long) lemon zest	1
½ cup	fresh or thawed frozen blueberries	125 mL
¼ cup	freshly squeezed lemon juice	50 mL
1½ cups	ice water or sparkling water	375 mL

1. In a small saucepan, bring sugar, the ¼ cup (50 mL) water and lemon zest to a boil. Reduce heat to low and simmer, uncovered, for 3 minutes. Remove lemon zest.

2. Transfer syrup to blender and add blueberries and lemon juice; purée on high speed.

3. Strain through a sieve into a large pitcher. Cover and refrigerate until cold. To serve, mix in ice water and pour into tall glasses.

Orange Cream Float

1 cup	fresh or drained canned mandarin orange sections	250 mL
1 cup	orange juice	250 mL
4 tsp	liquid honey	20 mL
1 tsp	vanilla	5 mL
2 cups	sparkling water	500 mL
1 cup	vanilla bean ice cream	250 mL

1. In blender, on high speed, purée orange, orange juice, honey and vanilla. Pour in sparkling water and pulse to blend. Pour into tall glasses and add ice cream.

Strawberry Soda Float

1⅓ cups	fresh or frozen strawberries	325 mL
2 tbsp	granulated sugar	25 mL
1 tsp	vanilla	5 mL
2 cups	sparkling water	500 mL
1 cup	strawberry ice cream	250 mL

1. In blender, on high speed, purée strawberries, sugar and vanilla. Pour in sparkling water and pulse to combine. Pour into tall glasses and add ice cream.

Sweet Lassi

1 cup	plain yogurt	250 mL
½ cup	water	125 mL
4 tsp	granulated sugar	20 mL
½ tsp	rose water	2 mL
Generous pinch	ground nutmeg	Generous pinch
Pinch	cayenne pepper	Pinch
4	ice cubes	4
2 tsp	finely chopped pistachios (optional)	10 mL

1. In blender, on high speed, blend yogurt, water, sugar, rose water, nutmeg, cayenne pepper and ice until smooth and frothy. Pour into chilled glasses and sprinkle with pistachios, if using.

An unusual, savory drink to cool down with on a hot summer day. Adjust salt to taste.

TIP

If you don't have cumin seeds, add 1/4 tsp (1 mL) ground cumin directly to blender.

Salty Lassi

1 tsp	cumin seeds (approx.)	5 mL
1 cup	plain yogurt	250 mL
1/2 cup	water	125 mL
2 tsp	freshly squeezed lemon juice	10 mL
1/2 tsp	salt (or to taste)	2 mL
4	ice cubes	4

1. In a dry heavy-bottomed skillet wiped clean of any lingering oil, over low heat, toast cumin seeds, shaking pan, for 2 to 3 minutes, or until fragrant and slightly darkened. Let cool and crush with a mortar and pestle or a spice grinder.

2. In blender, on high speed, blend yogurt, water, lemon juice, salt, crushed cumin and ice until smooth and frothy. Pour into chilled glasses and sprinkle with additional crushed cumin, if desired.

A delicious, savory starter or an accompaniment to spicy curries.

Tomato Lassi

1 cup	plain yogurt	250 mL
1 cup	tomato juice	250 mL
1/2 cup	water	125 mL
1/2 tsp	celery salt	2 mL
1/4 tsp	cayenne pepper	1 mL
4	ice cubes	4

1. In blender, on high speed, blend yogurt, tomato juice, water, celery salt, cayenne pepper and ice until smooth and frothy. Pour into chilled glasses.

Nonfat yogurt makes this a guilt-free drink for an afternoon refresher or an accompaniment to an Indian meal.

TIP

If you don't have cardamom seeds, add ¼ tsp (1 mL) ground cardamom directly to blender.

Mango Lassi

1 cup	nonfat plain yogurt	250 mL
1 cup	cubed peeled fresh mango or canned mango pulp	250 mL
8	cardamom pods, seeds only	8
½ cup	water	125 mL
2 tbsp	granulated sugar	25 mL
½ tsp	rose water	2 mL
4	ice cubes	4
2 tsp	finely chopped pistachios (optional)	10 mL

1. In blender, on high speed, purée yogurt and mango. Add cardamom seeds, water, sugar, rose water and ice; blend until well combined. Pour into chilled glasses and sprinkle with pistachios, if using.

Variation

Replace mango with other fruits, such as pineapple, papaya, strawberries, banana or a combination of tropical fruits.

Saffron gives this special drink a beautiful yellow color and perfumed aroma.

Saffron-Pistachio Lassi

¼ tsp	saffron threads	1 mL
2 tbsp	hot water	25 mL
8	cardamom pods, seeds only	8
3 tbsp	pistachios (approx.)	45 mL
2 tbsp	granulated sugar	25 mL
2 cups	milk	500 mL
4	ice cubes	4

1. In a small bowl, soak saffron in hot water for 10 minutes.

2. In blender, on high speed, purée cardamom seeds, pistachios and sugar. Add milk, ice and saffron with water; blend until smooth. Pour into chilled glasses and sprinkle with additional finely chopped pistachios, if desired.

A lovely summertime cooler or a complement to a Moroccan feast.

Moroccan Carrot Drink

1 cup	grated peeled carrot	250 mL
1 cup	orange juice	250 mL
1/4 cup	water	50 mL
2 tbsp	freshly squeezed lemon juice	25 mL
4 tsp	granulated sugar	20 mL

1. In blender, on high speed, purée carrot, orange juice, water, lemon juice and sugar. Pour into tall glasses, over ice.

The complementary flavors of celery, carrot and apple make this a juice bar favorite.

Carrot-Apple Drink

1 cup	grated peeled carrot	250 mL
1 cup	chopped celery	250 mL
1 cup	unsweetened apple juice	250 mL
1 cup	water	250 mL

1. In blender, on high speed, purée carrot, celery, apple juice and water. Strain through a fine sieve into tall glasses, over ice, if desired.

This sweet Caribbean drink is a treat with or without the rum.

Carrot Punch

8 cups	grated peeled carrots	2 L
4 cups	water, divided	1 L
2/3 cup	sweetened condensed milk	150 mL
1/4 tsp	ground nutmeg	1 mL
1 oz	rum (or to taste) (optional)	25 mL

1. In blender, on low speed, blend carrots and $1\frac{1}{2}$ cups (375 mL) of the water until very finely chopped. Squeeze with hands through a fine sieve or in cheesecloth to release enough juice to measure 1 cup (250 mL).

2. In same blender, on high speed, blend carrot juice, the remaining $2\frac{1}{2}$ cups (625 mL) water, condensed milk, nutmeg and rum (if using) until smooth. Pour into tall glasses, over ice.

Another favorite Caribbean drink, this one tastes like a peanut butter milkshake.

Peanut Punch

1 cup	evaporated milk	250 mL
1 cup	water	250 mL
1/4 cup	peanut butter	50 mL
3 tbsp	sweetened condensed milk (or to taste)	45 mL
1/4 tsp	ground nutmeg	1 mL
1/2 tsp	vanilla	2 mL

1. In blender, on high speed, blend evaporated milk, water, peanut butter, condensed milk, nutmeg and vanilla until smooth and creamy. Pour into tall glasses, over ice, if desired.

Variation

Peanut-Banana Punch: Add 1 very ripe banana.

This is an old Victorian pick-me-up and food for invalids, not to be confused with a cocktail.

This recipe contains raw eggs. If the food safety of raw eggs is a concern for you, use the pasteurized liquid whole egg instead.

Egg Flip

2	eggs (or 1/2 cup/125 mL pasteurized liquid whole egg)	2
1 1/2 cups	milk	375 mL
2 tbsp to 1/4 cup	sherry or white or red port	25 to 50 mL

1. In blender, on high speed, blend egg, milk and sherry until frothy.

Vanilla Rice Milk

Though rice milk is not a protein-rich drink like milk or soy milk, its lovely flavor and light texture make it perfect for lower-fat milkshakes.

2 cups	cooked brown rice	500 mL
3 cups	hot water, divided	750 mL
2 tbsp	pure maple syrup	25 mL
2 tsp	vanilla	10 mL

1. In blender, combine rice with 2 cups (500 mL) of the hot water. Let stand for 30 minutes, until softened. Add the remaining 1 cup (250 mL) hot water and blend on high speed until smooth. Strain through a fine sieve. Return to clean blender with maple syrup and vanilla; blend on high speed until smooth and creamy.

Variation

Homemade Rice Milk: Omit the vanilla.

Chocolate Rice Milk

2 cups	cooked brown rice	500 mL
3 cups	hot water, divided	750 mL
2 tbsp	boiling water	25 mL
4 tsp	unsweetened cocoa powder	20 mL
1/4 cup	pure maple syrup	50 mL
2 tsp	vanilla	10 mL

1. In blender, combine rice with 2 cups (500 mL) of the hot water. Let stand for 30 minutes, until softened. Add the remaining 1 cup (250 mL) hot water and blend on high speed until smooth. Strain through a fine sieve. Return to clean blender.

2. In a small bowl, stir together boiling water and cocoa to make a paste. Add to blender with maple syrup and vanilla; blend on high speed until smooth and creamy.

Soy Milk

Soy milk is readily available in many flavors, but it's also easy to make your own. Silken tofu is the best choice for blending as firmer varieties are too chunky to blend smoothly. Add a little more or less water to create the texture you desire.

8 oz	silken or soft tofu	250 g
1 cup	water (or to taste)	250 mL
4 tsp	pure maple syrup or light corn syrup (optional)	20 mL

1. In blender, on high speed, purée tofu, water and maple syrup (if using).

Variations

Vanilla Soy Milk: Add 2 tsp (10 mL) vanilla.

Chocolate Soy Milk: Mix 4 tsp (20 mL) unsweetened cocoa powder with 2 tbsp (25 mL) boiling water and add to blender. Increase syrup to $1/4$ cup (50 mL).

Soy Breakfast Blend

A quick and easy start to the day. Frozen punch concentrate adds a little extra kick; look for a pineapple-orange punch for the best flavor.

1	banana	1
1 cup	fresh or frozen strawberries	250 mL
1 cup	plain or vanilla-flavored soy milk	250 mL
3 tbsp	frozen pineapple-orange or orange punch concentrate	45 mL
8	ice cubes	8

1. In blender, on high speed, blend banana, strawberries, soy milk, pineapple-orange punch concentrate and ice until smooth and creamy.

A sweet and tasty alternative to that second cup of morning coffee. Slightly black and soft (but not squishy) bananas give the best flavor.

TIP

For this drink, brew coffee very strong or mix 2 tsp (10 mL) instant coffee granules with 1/3 cup (75 mL) boiling water. Let cool to room temperature before using.

Frozen Banana-Soy Latte

1	banana	1
1 cup	plain or vanilla-flavored soy milk	250 mL
2/3 cup	cooled very strong coffee (see tip, at left)	150 mL
6	ice cubes	6
1/4 tsp	unsweetened cocoa powder or ground cinnamon	1 mL

1. In blender, on high speed, purée banana, soy milk, coffee and ice. Pour into a glass and sprinkle with cocoa.

TIP

To make your own Chai tea blend: In an airtight container, combine 1 cup (250 mL) black tea leaves (such as Darjeeling or orange pekoe), 6 bay leaves, broken, 24 whole cloves, 24 whole black peppercorns, 12 green cardamom pods, broken, and 3 cinnamon sticks, broken. Makes 1 1/4 cups (300 mL).

Chai Latte

2/3 cup	milk or soy milk	150 mL
2/3 cup	water	150 mL
2 tbsp	granulated sugar (or to taste)	25 mL
2 tbsp	loose Chai tea blend (or 1 Chai tea bag)	25 mL

1. In a small saucepan, combine milk, water and sugar. Add tea and bring to a simmer. Remove from heat and let steep for 5 minutes. Return just to a boil, remove from heat and let rest for 1 minute.

2. Strain tea into blender and blend on high speed until frothy.

MAKES 2 SERVINGS

MAKES 2 SERVINGS

You don't need a fancy espresso machine to enjoy cappuccino on Sunday mornings. Brew double-strength coffee (preferably with espresso or French roast beans) and froth hot milk in the blender.

TIP

Blend only ⅔ cup (150 mL) hot milk at a time — it needs room to foam inside the blender. It's a good idea to secure the lid with a thick dish towel in case of spillage.

Blender Cappuccino

1 ⅓ cups	milk or soy milk	325 mL
⅔ cup	hot strong brewed coffee	150 mL
Generous pinch	ground cinnamon or unsweetened cocoa powder (optional)	Generous pinch

1. In a small saucepan, bring milk to a boil. Remove from heat and let stand for 1 minute.

2. Transfer to blender and blend on high speed until frothy.

3. Pour coffee into a large warm cup or mug. Using a spoon to hold back foam, pour in hot foamy milk to coffee. Scoop light foam on top. Sprinkle with cinnamon, if using.

Variations

Caffé Latte: Pour coffee into a large warm mug or bowl. Pour foamed milk into coffee. Sprinkle with cinnamon or unsweetened cocoa powder, if desired.

Mochaccino: Blend 2 tbsp (25 mL) chocolate syrup (or to taste) with the hot milk. Prepare as for cappuccino.

MAKES 2 SERVINGS

Made popular by coffee chains, iced coffee drinks are very easy (and more economical) to make at home. Add 1 tbsp (15 mL) flavored syrup, such as almond, mint or orange, for an extra kick.

Iced Coffee Frappé

1 ⅓ cups	cold double-strength brewed coffee	325 mL
½ cup	half-and-half (10%) cream or milk	125 mL
2 tbsp	granulated sugar	25 mL

1. Pour coffee into an ice cube tray and freeze until firm, about 4 hours.

2. In blender, on high speed, blend coffee cubes, cream and sugar until slushy. Pour into a chilled glass.

Variation

Mochaccino: Replace cream with chocolate milk and reduce sugar to taste.

Vietnamese restaurants are known for strong coffee filtered over ice and sweetened condensed milk. This blended version is the ultimate coffee frappé. French roasts or coffees with chicory (like Café du Monde) give the most authentic taste.

Blended Vietnamese Iced Coffee

1 ½ cups	very strong coffee, cooled	375 mL
2 tbsp	sweetened condensed milk (or to taste)	25 mL
8	ice cubes	8

1. In blender, on high speed, blend coffee, condensed milk and ice until smooth and slushy. Pour into a chilled glass.

Mexican chocolate tablets are sold in round discs; you just break off a piece and blend with hot milk for a creamy, frothy drink. This method yields similar results.

TIP

This recipe multiplies easily for several servings, but blend only ¾ cup (175 mL) hot milk mixture at a time, as it needs room to foam inside the blender. It's a good idea to secure the lid with a thick dish towel in case of spillage.

Mexican Hot Chocolate

2 cups	milk	500 mL
2 oz	semi-sweet chocolate, chopped	60 g
4 tsp	granulated sugar	20 mL
½ tsp	vanilla	2 mL
¼ tsp	ground cinnamon	1 mL
1	drop almond extract (optional)	1

1. In a small saucepan, combine milk, chocolate, sugar, vanilla, cinnamon and almond extract (if using). Bring to a simmer over medium-low heat and simmer gently for 1 to 2 minutes, or until chocolate is melted.

2. Transfer to blender and blend on high speed until smooth and frothy.

Cocktails

Alcohol is traditionally measured in ounces. Shot glasses are 2-ounce measures, often marked with 1- and 1½-ounce measures. One ounce equals 2 tablespoons (25 mL); 2 ounces equals ¼ cup (50 mL). Always rinse out your shot glass and blender between cocktails.

Blenders have always been indispensable bar tools and the new generation of blenders have the power to chop ice with ease, allowing you to make wonderful slushy or chilled drinks. Standard cocktails, such as martinis or manhattans, tend to become too watered down when blended, so if you want to improvise, stick to drinks — like those in this book — that use the blender to purée fruit, make frothy drinks or smooth ice cream into a cocktail. Frozen fruit concentrates are an excellent choice, as they combine with ice to chill and not dilute your cocktail. Experimenting with seasonal fruits is fun. Gather friends for a blender cocktail contest (good friends of mine hold an annual contest at a summer barbecue). Be daring — you might invent the perfect blender drink.

MAKES 2 CUPS (500 ML)

Simple Syrup is used in some of the cocktails.

Simple Syrup

1 cup	granulated sugar	250 mL
1 cup	water	250 mL

1. In a small saucepan, bring sugar and water to a boil. Boil until sugar is dissolved. Let cool.

2. *Make ahead:* Pour into a sealable jar or an airtight container. Seal and store at room temperature for up to 1 week.

This famous Jamaican drink blends sweet milk with bitter stout for a drink that tastes a little like a Chai milkshake.

Guinness Punch

¼ cup	sweetened condensed milk	50 mL
Pinch	ground nutmeg	Pinch
Pinch	ground cinnamon	Pinch
Pinch	unsweetened cocoa powder (optional)	Pinch
1 cup	stout (such as Guinness)	250 mL

1. In blender, on high speed, blend condensed milk, nutmeg, cinnamon, cocoa (if using) and stout until smooth and well combined. Pour into a chilled glass.

Cuban Punch

½ tsp	freshly grated orange zest	2 mL
1 cup	orange juice	250 mL
½ cup	frozen strawberries	125 mL
½ cup	cubed pineapple	125 mL
2 oz	coconut or amber rum	50 mL
1	ice cube	1

1. In blender, on high speed, blend orange zest, orange juice, strawberries, pineapple, rum and ice until smooth. Pour into a large stemmed punch glass.

Shark Attack

¼ cup	frozen orange juice concentrate	50 mL
4 tsp	freshly squeezed lime juice	20 mL
2 oz	amber rum	50 mL
½ oz	orange liqueur	15 mL
4	ice cubes	4
1 tbsp	grenadine	15 mL

1. In blender, on high speed, blend orange juice concentrate, lime juice, rum, orange liqueur and ice until slushy. Pour into a highball glass and top with grenadine.

All over Taiwan, non-alcoholic papaya shakes are for sale. Why not spike it up?

Taiwan Papaya Shake

1 cup	cubed peeled and seeded papaya	250 mL
3 tbsp	sweetened condensed milk	45 mL
1 tsp	freshly squeezed lime juice	5 mL
2 oz	white or amber rum	50 mL
3	ice cubes	3

1. In blender, on high speed, blend papaya, milk, lime juice, rum and ice until smooth. Pour into a tall glass.

Cranberry Cooler

¼ cup	frozen cranberry cocktail concentrate	50 mL
2 oz	white rum	50 mL
1 oz	orange liqueur	25 mL
6	ice cubes	6
¼ cup	tonic water	50 mL
1	lime wedge	1

1. In blender, on high speed, blend cranberry cocktail concentrate, rum, orange liqueur and ice until smooth. Pour into a highball glass and top with tonic water. Garnish with lime wedge.

Tomahawk

2 tbsp	frozen cranberry cocktail concentrate	25 mL
2 tbsp	frozen pineapple juice concentrate	25 mL
2 oz	white or amber rum	50 mL
½ oz	orange liqueur	15 mL
6	ice cubes	6
1	lime wedge	1

1. In blender, on high speed, blend cranberry cocktail and pineapple juice concentrates, rum, orange liqueur and ice until smooth. Pour into an old-fashioned glass and garnish with lime wedge.

Bananarama

½	banana	½
2 tbsp	freshly squeezed lime juice	25 mL
1 ½ tsp	confectioner's (icing) sugar	7 mL
2 oz	white, amber or dark rum	50 mL
3	ice cubes	3

1. In blender, on high speed, blend banana, lime juice, sugar, rum and ice until smooth. Pour into a highball glass.

Bee's Bananarama

½	banana	½
1 tbsp	liquid honey	15 mL
2 tsp	freshly squeezed lemon juice	10 mL
1 oz	white or amber rum	25 mL
1 oz	brandy	25 mL
3	ice cubes	3
Pinch	ground cinnamon	Pinch

1. In blender, on high speed, blend banana, honey, lemon juice, rum, brandy and ice until smooth. Pour into a highball glass and sprinkle with cinnamon.

Jamaican Dirty Banana

½	banana	½
¼ cup	table (18%) cream	50 mL
1 ½ oz	amber or dark Jamaican rum	40 mL
1 oz	coffee liqueur, such as Kahlúa	25 mL
1 oz	crème de banane	25 mL
3	ice cubes	3

1. In blender, on high speed, blend banana, cream, rum, coffee liqueur, crème de banane and ice until smooth. Pour into a highball glass.

Tiger Stripes

2 tbsp	chocolate syrup	25 mL
½	banana	½
1 cup	milk	250 mL
1½ oz	amber rum	40 mL
5	ice cubes	5

1. Drizzle chocolate syrup into a chilled highball glass, rotating glass as you drizzle to form a spiral.

2. In blender, on high speed, blend banana, milk, rum and ice until smooth. Pour into glass.

Coconut Rum Punch

½ cup	coconut milk	125 mL
2 tsp	palm sugar or light brown sugar	10 mL
1 tsp	freshly squeezed lime juice	5 mL
2 oz	amber rum	50 mL
2	ice cubes	2

1. In blender, on high speed, blend coconut milk, sugar, lime juice, rum and ice cubes until smooth. Pour into a large stemmed punch glass or coconut shell.

For a real multo-buko, replace the coconut milk with 1 cup (250 mL) fresh young coconut (buko in Tagalog), including its gelatinous flesh.

Mock Multo-Buko

½ cup	coconut milk	125 mL
1 tbsp	freshly squeezed lime juice	15 mL
1 tbsp	Simple Syrup (see recipe, page 237)	15 mL
2 oz	amber rum	50 mL
6	ice cubes	6
1	slice lime	1

1. In blender, on high speed, blend coconut milk, lime juice, syrup, rum and ice until smooth. Pour into a large highball glass or coconut shell and garnish with lime slice.

Piña Colada

MAKES 1 SERVING

Creamed coconut is already sweetened. If you use coconut milk, use ¼ cup (50 mL) from the top of the can (the coconut cream) and add 1 tbsp (15 mL) Simple Syrup (see recipe, page 237).

1 cup	cubed pineapple	250 mL
2 tbsp	creamed coconut	25 mL
1½ oz	amber or white rum	40 mL
3	ice cubes	3
1	lime wedge (optional)	1

1. In blender, on high speed, blend pineapple, creamed coconut, rum and ice until smooth. Pour into a highball glass and garnish with lime wedge, if desired.

MAKES 1 SERVING

Trinidad Piña Colada

1 cup	cubed pineapple	250 mL
2 tbsp	creamed coconut	25 mL
Pinch	salt	Pinch
1½ oz	amber or white rum	40 mL
4 dashes	angostura bitters	4 dashes
3	ice cubes	3

1. In blender, on high speed, blend pineapple, creamed coconut, salt, rum, bitters and ice until smooth. Pour into a highball glass.

MAKES 1 SERVING

Aqua Piña Colada

1 cup	cubed pineapple	250 mL
2 tbsp	creamed coconut	25 mL
2 tsp	freshly squeezed lime juice	10 mL
1½ oz	amber or white rum	40 mL
1 oz	blue curaçao	25 mL
3	ice cubes	3

1. In blender, on high speed, blend pineapple, creamed coconut, lime juice, rum, blue curaçao and ice until smooth. Pour into a highball glass.

Strawberry Colada

12	fresh or frozen strawberries	12
2 tbsp	creamed coconut	25 mL
2 tbsp	vanilla ice cream	25 mL
2 oz	amber or white rum	50 mL
3	ice cubes	3
1	lemon or lime wedge (optional)	1

1. In blender, on high speed, blend strawberries, creamed coconut, ice cream, rum and ice until smooth. Pour into a highball glass and garnish with lemon wedge, if desired.

Pink Piña

1 cup	unsweetened pineapple juice	250 mL
3 tbsp	coconut cream	45 mL
2 tbsp	strawberry syrup	25 mL
1 1/2 oz	amber rum	40 mL
5	ice cubes	5
1	strawberry (optional)	1

1. In blender, on high speed, blend pineapple juice, coconut cream, strawberry syrup, rum and ice until smooth. Pour into a highball glass and garnish with strawberry, if desired.

Pilipino Piña

1/2 cup	cubed pineapple	125 mL
2 tsp	cane syrup or Simple Syrup (see recipe, page 237)	10 mL
2 tsp	freshly squeezed lime juice	10 mL
2 oz	amber rum	50 mL
4	ice cubes	4

1. In blender, on high speed, blend pineapple, syrup, lime juice, rum and ice until smooth. Pour into a highball glass.

Frozen Daiquiri

2	ice cubes	2
2 tbsp	freshly squeezed lime juice	25 mL
1 tsp	confectioner's (icing) sugar	5 mL
2 oz	white rum	50 mL

1. In blender, pulse ice until crushed. On high speed, blend in lime juice, sugar and rum until slushy. Pour into an old-fashioned or martini glass.

Frozen Berry Daiquiri

1	ice cube	1
6	frozen strawberries	6
2 tbsp	freshly squeezed lime juice	25 mL
2 tsp	strawberry syrup	10 mL
2 oz	white rum	50 mL

1. In blender, pulse ice and strawberries until ice is crushed. On high speed, blend in lime juice, strawberry syrup and rum until slushy. Pour into an old-fashioned or martini glass.

TIP

To peel a fresh peach, submerge it in boiling water for 10 to 15 seconds to loosen the skin. Or use drained canned peaches or frozen peaches.

Frozen Peach Daiquiri

2	ice cubes	2
1/2 cup	cubed peeled peaches (see tip, at left)	125 mL
2 tbsp	freshly squeezed lime juice	25 mL
1 1/2 tsp	confectioner's (icing) sugar	7 mL
2 oz	white rum	50 mL
1 oz	peach schnapps	25 mL

1. In blender, pulse ice and peach until ice is crushed. On high speed, blend in lime juice, sugar, rum and peach schnapps until slushy. Pour into an old-fashioned or martini glass.

Frozen Lichee Daiquiri

2	ice cubes	2
5	canned lichees, drained	5
2 tbsp	freshly squeezed lime juice	25 mL
2 tsp	syrup from canned lichees	10 mL
2 oz	white rum	50 mL

1. In blender, pulse ice and lichees until ice is crushed. On high speed, blend in lime juice, syrup and rum until slushy. Pour into an old-fashioned or martini glass.

Frozen Coconut Daiquiri

2	ice cubes	2
2 tbsp	freshly squeezed lime juice	25 mL
2 tsp	creamed coconut	10 mL
1 1/2 oz	white rum	40 mL
1 oz	coconut rum	25 mL

1. In blender, pulse ice until crushed. On high speed, blend in lime juice, creamed coconut, and white and coconut rums until slushy. Pour into an old-fashioned or martini glass.

Frozen Banana Daiquiri

3	ice cubes	3
1/2	banana	1/2
2 tbsp	freshly squeezed lime juice	25 mL
2 oz	white rum	50 mL
1 oz	crème de banane	25 mL

1. In blender, pulse ice and banana until ice is crushed. On high speed, blend in lime juice, rum and crème de banane until slushy. Pour into an old-fashioned or martini glass.

This warming (and nutritious) winter drink is much easier to make in the blender than with the traditional whisking method.

This recipe contains a raw egg. If the food safety of raw eggs is a concern for you, use the pasteurized liquid whole egg instead.

Tom and Jerry

1	egg, separated (or ¼ cup/50 mL pasteurized liquid whole egg)	1
1 tbsp	confectioner's (icing) sugar	15 mL
1½ oz	dark rum	40 mL
1½ oz	brandy	40 mL
½ cup	boiling water (approx.)	125 mL
Pinch	freshly ground nutmeg	Pinch

1. In blender, on high speed, beat egg white until frothy. Add yolk and continue blending until very frothy. (Or blend pasteurized liquid whole egg until very frothy.) Blend in rum and brandy just until mixed. Pour into a mug and top with boiling water. Sprinkle with nutmeg.

This recipe contains a raw egg yolk. If the food safety of raw eggs is a concern for you, use the pasteurized liquid whole egg instead.

Easy Eggnog

1	egg yolk (or 2 tbsp/25 mL pasteurized liquid whole egg)	1
¼ cup	whipping (35%) cream	50 mL
2 tsp	liquid honey	10 mL
2 oz	brandy or dark rum	50 mL
4	ice cubes	4
Pinch	freshly ground nutmeg	Pinch

1. In blender, on high speed, blend egg yolk, whipping cream, honey, brandy and ice until smooth. Pour into an eggnog cup or a punch cup and sprinkle with nutmeg.

Tofu Eggnog

½ cup	silken or soft tofu	125 mL
¼ cup	water	50 mL
3 tbsp	packed soft brown sugar	45 mL
½ tsp	vanilla	2 mL
¼ tsp	ground turmeric	1 mL
¼ tsp	ground nutmeg (approx.)	1 mL
1 oz	rum or brandy (or to taste)	25 mL

1. In blender, on high speed, blend tofu, water, sugar, vanilla, turmeric, nutmeg and rum until smooth and creamy. Pour into a glass and sprinkle with additional nutmeg, if desired.

This recipe contains raw egg yolks. If the food safety of raw eggs is a concern for you, use the pasteurized liquid whole egg instead. The 'nog will not thicken as much, but you can add some vanilla ice cream to give a thicker consistency, if desired.

Shooter 'Nog

6	egg yolks (or ⅔ cup/150 mL pasteurized liquid whole egg)	6
½ cup	granulated sugar	125 mL
1½ tsp	vanilla	7 mL
½ tsp	ground nutmeg	2 mL
13 oz	vodka (about ½ bottle)	375 mL
3 oz	cognac or other brandy	75 mL
1½ oz	Scotch whisky	40 mL

1. In blender, on high speed, blend egg yolks and sugar until creamy. Blend in vanilla, nutmeg, vodka, brandy and Scotch until smooth. Pour into a freezer-proof bottle or container and store in the freezer for up to 1 month.

MAKES 1 SERVING

If you love pomegranates, you'll love this cocktail!

Pomegranate Cocktail

¼ cup	pomegranate seeds	50 mL
1 tsp	freshly squeezed lime juice	5 mL
½ tsp	confectioner's (icing) sugar	2 mL
1 oz	vodka	25 mL

1. In blender, on high speed, blend pomegranate seeds, lime juice, sugar and vodka until pomegranate flesh is separated from seed cores. Strain through a fine sieve into an old-fashioned glass filled with ice.

MAKES 1 SERVING

Pom Pilot

¼ cup	pomegranate seeds	50 mL
1 oz	orange liqueur	25 mL
1 oz	brandy	25 mL

1. In blender, on high speed, blend pomegranate seeds, orange liqueur and brandy until pomegranate flesh is separated from seed cores. Strain through a fine sieve into an old-fashioned glass filled with ice.

MAKES 1 SERVING

Pom-Pom

¼ cup	pomegranate seeds	50 mL
¼ cup	orange juice	50 mL
1 tsp	freshly squeezed lemon juice	5 mL
½ tsp	confectioner's (icing) sugar	2 mL
1½ oz	vodka	40 mL

1. In blender, on high speed, blend pomegranate seeds, orange and lemon juices, sugar and vodka until pomegranate flesh is separated from seed cores. Strain through a fine sieve into a highball glass filled with ice.

Frozen Rush Hour

1 ½ tsp	blackcurrant concentrate (such as Ribena)	7 mL
1 oz	vodka	25 mL
1 oz	red vermouth	25 mL
¼ oz	cherry brandy	7 mL
2	ice cubes	2

1. In blender, on high speed, blend blackcurrant concentrate, vodka, vermouth, cherry brandy and ice until smooth. Pour into an old-fashioned or martini glass.

Frosty Screwdriver

¼ cup	frozen orange juice concentrate	50 mL
2 oz	vodka	50 mL
½ oz	orange liqueur	15 mL
6	ice cubes	6
1	slice orange	1

1. In blender, on high speed, blend orange juice concentrate, vodka, orange liqueur and ice until smooth. Pour into a highball glass and garnish with orange slice.

Mama's Mango

½	mango, peeled and cubed	½
1 tbsp	freshly squeezed lime juice	15 mL
1 tsp	confectioner's (icing) sugar	5 mL
1 oz	vodka	25 mL
½ oz	orange liqueur	15 mL
4	ice cubes	4

1. In blender, on high speed, blend mango, lime juice, sugar, vodka, orange liqueur and ice until smooth. Pour into an old-fashioned or large stemmed punch glass.

Minty Pineapple Spritz

6	fresh mint leaves (or generous dash white crème de menthe)	6
½ cup	cubed pineapple	125 mL
1 tsp	confectioner's (icing) sugar	5 mL
1 tsp	freshly squeezed lemon juice	5 mL
1 oz	vodka	25 mL
¼ cup	soda water or seltzer	50 mL

1. In blender, on high speed, blend mint, pineapple, sugar, lemon juice and vodka until smooth. Pour into a large highball glass filled with ice and top with soda.

Lichee Lust

4	canned lichees, drained	4
1 tbsp	syrup from canned lichees	15 mL
1 tsp	freshly squeezed lime juice	5 mL
1 oz	brandy	25 mL
2	ice cubes	2
Dash	grenadine	Dash

1. In blender, on high speed, blend lichees, syrup, lime juice, brandy and ice until smooth. Pour into an old-fashioned glass and top with grenadine.

Use only unsprayed fragrant rose petals.

TIP

If rose petals are not available, substitute ¼ tsp (1 mL) rose water (no need to strain).

Gypsy Rose

¼ cup	loosely packed rose petals	50 mL
2 oz	vodka	50 mL
1 tsp	grenadine	5 mL
2	ice cubes	2

1. In blender, on high speed, blend rose petals, vodka, grenadine and ice until rose petals and ice are finely chopped. Strain through a fine sieve into a martini glass.

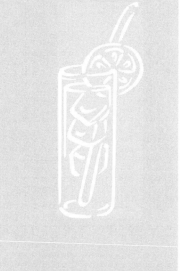

Sparkling Blackcurrant Lemonade

2 tbsp	frozen lemonade concentrate	25 mL
2 oz	vodka	50 mL
1 oz	crème de cassis	25 mL
6	ice cubes	6
¼ cup	soda water or seltzer	50 mL
1	slice lemon	1

1. In blender, on high speed, blend lemonade concentrate, vodka, crème de cassis and ice until smooth. Pour into a highball glass and top with soda water. Garnish with lemon slice.

You can omit the hot peppers if you use chili pepper vodka instead of regular vodka. Hot pepper lovers should use both.

Hot Honeydew Freezie

1 cup	cubed very ripe honeydew melon	250 mL
2 tbsp	freshly squeezed lime juice	25 mL
1½ tsp	confectioner's (icing) sugar	7 mL
1 tsp	chopped seeded green hot pepper	5 mL
Pinch	salt	Pinch
1½ oz	vodka or chili pepper vodka	40 mL
½ oz	orange liqueur	15 mL
6	ice cubes	6

1. In blender, on high speed, blend , lime juice, sugar, hot pepper, salt, vodka, orange liqueur and ice until smooth. Pour into a highball or large stemmed punch glass.

You can omit the hot peppers if you use chili pepper vodka instead of regular vodka. Hot pepper lovers should use both.

Hot Watermelon Freezie

1 cup	cubed seedless watermelon	250 mL
1 tbsp	freshly squeezed lemon juice	25 mL
1 tsp	confectioner's (icing) sugar	5 mL
1 tsp	chopped seeded red hot pepper	5 mL
Pinch	salt	Pinch
1½ oz	vodka or chili pepper vodka	40 mL
½ oz	orange liqueur	15 mL
6	ice cubes	6

1. In blender, on high speed, blend melon, lemon juice, sugar, hot pepper, salt, vodka, orange liqueur and ice until smooth. Pour into a highball or large stemmed punch glass.

Hot Pink Ginger

1 tbsp	freshly squeezed lime juice	15 mL
2 tsp	chopped ginger in syrup or pickled ginger	10 mL
1 tsp	grenadine	5 mL
2 oz	vodka	50 mL
2	ice cubes	2

1. In blender, on high speed, blend lime juice, ginger, grenadine, vodka and ice until smooth. Pour into a martini glass.

Winter Whippet

¼ cup	frozen grapefruit juice concentrate	50 mL
2 oz	vodka	50 mL
6	ice cubes	6

1. In blender, on high speed, blend grapefruit juice concentrate, vodka and ice until slushy. Pour into a highball glass.

Pink Whippet

¼ cup	frozen pink grapefruit juice concentrate	50 mL
1 tsp	grenadine	5 mL
2 oz	vodka	50 mL
2 dashes	angostura bitters	2 dashes
6	ice cubes	6

1. In blender, on high speed, blend grapefruit juice concentrate, grenadine, vodka, bitters and ice until slushy. Pour into an old-fashioned glass.

Sweeter than a regular cosmo, but balanced with a little lime juice, this is a refreshing summer cocktail.

Frozen Cosmo

3	ice cubes	3
1 tbsp	frozen cranberry cocktail concentrate	15 mL
2 tsp	freshly squeezed lime juice	10 mL
2 oz	vodka	50 mL
1 oz	orange brandy or orange liqueur	25 mL
1 to 3	frozen cranberries (optional)	1 to 3

1. In blender, pulse ice until crushed. On high speed, blend in cranberry cocktail concentrate, lime juice, vodka and orange brandy until slushy. Pour into a martini glass and garnish with frozen cranberries, if desired.

Watermelon Cosmo

1 cup	cubed seedless watermelon, frozen	250 mL
2 tbsp	cranberry cocktail	25 mL
4 tsp	freshly squeezed lime juice	20 mL
1 ½ oz	vodka or citrus vodka	40 mL
½ oz	melon liqueur	15 mL
2 dashes	angostura bitters	2 dashes

1. In blender, on high speed, blend watermelon, cranberry cocktail, lime juice, vodka, melon liqueur and bitters until smooth. Strain through a fine sieve into a martini glass.

La Vie en Rose

1 tbsp	freshly squeezed lemon juice	15 mL
1 tbsp	grenadine	15 mL
1 oz	vodka or gin	25 mL
1 oz	kirsch	25 mL
2	ice cubes	2
1	unsprayed rose petal (optional)	1

1. In blender, on high speed, blend lemon juice, grenadine, vodka, kirsch and ice until ice is well crushed. Pour into an old-fashioned glass and garnish with rose petal, if desired.

Green Goddess

6	fresh basil leaves	6
2 oz	gin or vodka	50 mL
1 oz	dry white vermouth	25 mL
1	ice cube	1
1	small black olive	1

1. In blender, on high speed, blend basil, gin, vermouth and ice until smooth. Strain through a fine sieve into a martini glass and garnish with olive.

Winter Greyhound

¼ cup	frozen grapefruit juice concentrate	50 mL
2 oz	gin	50 mL
6	ice cubes	6

1. In blender, on high speed, blend grapefruit juice concentrate, gin and ice until slushy. Pour into a highball glass.

Pink Greyhound

¼ cup	frozen pink grapefruit juice concentrate	50 mL
2 oz	gin	50 mL
2 dashes	angostura bitters	2 dashes
6	ice cubes	6

1. In blender, on high speed, blend grapefruit juice concentrate, gin, bitters and ice until slushy. Pour into a highball glass.

Pink Gin Whizz

1 tsp	confectioner's (icing) sugar	5 mL
1 tsp	freshly squeezed lemon juice	5 mL
2 oz	gin	50 mL
4 dashes	angostura bitters	4 dashes
2	ice cubes	2

1. In blender, on high speed, blend icing sugar, lemon juice, gin, bitters and ice until ice is well crushed. Pour into an old-fashioned glass.

For a version of this drink that is more like a digestive — perfect after a meal of oysters — add a few dashes of angostura bitters. This drink can also be called a Tom Collins Slushy.

Après les Huîtres

2 tbsp	frozen lemonade concentrate	25 mL
1 tbsp	Simple Syrup (see recipe, page 237)	15 mL
2 oz	gin	50 mL
1	ice cube	1
¼ cup	soda water or seltzer	50 mL
1	lemon wedge	1

1. In blender, on high speed, blend lemonade concentrate, Simple Syrup, gin and ice until smooth. Pour into a highball glass and top with soda. Garnish with lemon wedge.

Summer Pimm's Slushy

¼ cup	chopped peeled and seeded cucumber	50 mL
2 tsp	freshly squeezed lemon juice	10 mL
2 oz	Pimm's No. 1 liqueur	50 mL
2	ice cubes	2
¼ cup	soda water or seltzer	50 mL
1	slice lemon	1

1. In blender, on high speed, blend cucumber, lemon juice, Pimm's and ice until slushy but not altogether smooth. Pour into a highball glass and top with soda. Garnish with lemon slice.

Watermelon Martini

⅓ cup	cubed seedless watermelon, chilled	75 mL
Pinch	salt	Pinch
2 oz	vodka or gin	50 mL
1	ice cube	1

1. In blender, on high speed, blend watermelon, salt, vodka and ice until smooth. Pour into a martini glass.

Raspberry Martini

¼ cup	frozen unsweetened raspberries	50 mL
2 oz	gin or vodka	50 mL
1 oz	orange liqueur	25 mL
2 dashes	angostura bitters	2 dashes

1. In blender, on high speed, blend raspberries, gin, orange liqueur and bitters until smooth. Strain through a fine sieve into a martini glass.

Strawberry Pepper Martini

6	frozen strawberries	6
6	whole black peppercorns	6
3 oz	vodka	75 mL
Dash	orange liqueur	Dash

1. In blender, on high speed, blend strawberries, peppercorns, vodka and orange liqueur until strawberries are puréed and peppercorns are coarsely crushed. Pour into a martini glass.

Watermelon and Basil Martini

5	fresh basil leaves	5
1 cup	cubed seedless watermelon, frozen	250 mL
Pinch	salt	Pinch
2 oz	gin	50 mL
Dash	angostura bitters	Dash

1. In blender, on high speed, blend basil, watermelon, salt, gin and bitters until smooth. Strain through a fine sieve into a martini glass.

Essence of Pear Martini

¼ cup	cubed peeled very ripe pear	50 mL
1½ oz	poire Williams liqueur	40 mL
1	ice cube	1

1. In blender, on high speed, blend pear, poire Williams and ice until smooth. Pour into a martini glass.

Essence of Plum Martini

1	red or prune plum or pluot, peeled, halved and pitted	1
1 1/2 oz	plum eau-de-vie (such as Slivovitch or pruneaux or pflümli)	40 mL
1	ice cube	1

1. In blender, on high speed, blend plum, plum eau-de-vie and ice until smooth. Pour into a martini glass.

Essence of Cherry Martini

1/4 cup	pitted sweet cherries	50 mL
1 1/2 oz	kirsch	40 mL
1	ice cube	1

1. In blender, on high speed, blend cherries, kirsch and ice until smooth. Pour into a martini glass.

Essence of Apricot Martini

1	very ripe apricot, peeled, halved and pitted, or drained canned apricot	1
1 1/2 oz	apricot brandy	40 mL
1	ice cube	1

1. In blender, on high speed, blend apricot, apricot brandy and ice until smooth. Pour into a martini glass.

Piña Colada Martini

⅓ cup	cubed pineapple	75 mL
1 tsp	freshly squeezed lime juice	5 mL
2 oz	coconut rum	50 mL
1	ice cube	1

1. In blender, on high speed, blend pineapple, lime juice, coconut rum and ice until smooth. Pour into a martini glass.

Tutti Frutti Martini

2 tbsp	unsweetened apple juice	25 mL
2 tbsp	unsweetened pineapple juice	25 mL
1½ tsp	freshly squeezed lime juice	7 mL
1½ oz	raspberry vodka or citrus vodka	40 mL
½ oz	melon liqueur	25 mL
½ oz	peach schnapps	25 mL
1	ice cube	1
1	small wedge fresh pineapple, apple, peach or lime	1

1. In blender, on high speed, blend apple, pineapple and lime juices, vodka, melon liqueur, peach schnapps and ice until smooth. Pour into a martini glass and garnish with fruit.

Nutty Cream Martini

2 tbsp	vanilla ice cream	25 mL
2 oz	vodka	50 mL
1 oz	almond or hazelnut liqueur	25 mL
1	ice cube	1

1. In blender, on high speed, blend ice cream, vodka, almond liqueur and ice until smooth. Pour into a martini glass or a wide-mouthed champagne glass.

Vanilla Vanilla Cream Martini

2 tbsp	vanilla ice cream	25 mL
2½ oz	vanilla vodka	65 mL
½ oz	orange liqueur	15 mL
1	ice cube	1
1	small piece vanilla bean	1

1. In blender, on high speed, blend ice cream, vodka, orange liqueur and ice until smooth. Pour into a martini glass and garnish with vanilla bean.

Lemon Grass Martini

2 tbsp	chopped lemon grass (white part only)	25 mL
2 oz	vodka	50 mL
1 oz	dry white vermouth	25 mL
1	ice cube	1

1. In blender, on high speed, blend lemon grass, vodka, vermouth and ice until lemon grass is very finely chopped. Strain through a fine sieve into a martini glass.

Cuc'a Sake Martini

¼ cup	chopped peeled and seeded cucumber	50 mL
1 tsp	freshly squeezed lemon juice	5 mL
3 oz	sake	75 mL
1	ice cube	1
	Twist of cucumber peel	

1. In blender, on high speed, blend cucumber, lemon juice, sake and ice until smooth. Pour into a martini glass and garnish with cucumber peel.

Hamlet's Blood

1	pickled baby beet, drained	1
2 oz	frozen aquavit	50 mL

1. In blender, on high speed, blend beet and aquavit until smooth. Pour into a large shot glass.

Poseidon's Wave

2 tsp	freshly squeezed lemon juice	10 mL
2 oz	ouzo	50 mL
1/2 oz	dry white vermouth	15 mL
2	ice cubes	2
2	anchovy-stuffed olives	2

1. In blender, on high speed, blend lemon juice, ouzo, vermouth and ice until smooth. Pour into a martini glass. Thread olives onto a cocktail stick and plunge into drink.

Mock Gewürztraminer

4	canned lichees, drained	4
1 tbsp	syrup from canned lichees	15 mL
Dash	rose water	Dash
Dash	freshly squeezed lemon juice	Dash
3 oz	dry white vermouth	75 mL
2	ice cubes	2

1. In blender, on high speed, blend lichees, syrup, rose water, lemon juice, vermouth and ice cubes until smooth. Pour into a wine glass.

This recipe contains a raw egg white. If the food safety of raw eggs is a concern for you, use the pasteurized liquid egg white instead.

Gin Fizz

1	egg white (or 2 tbsp/25 mL pasteurized liquid egg white)	1
2 tbsp	freshly squeezed lemon juice	25 mL
1 tbsp	whipping (35%) cream	15 mL
1½ tsp	confectioner's (icing) sugar	7 mL
2 oz	gin	50 mL
2	ice cubes	2
2 tbsp	soda water or seltzer (approx.)	25 mL

1. In blender, on high speed, blend egg white, lemon juice, whipping cream, sugar, gin and ice until smooth and frothy. Pour into a highball glass and top with soda.

When blended, pineapple fizzes — almost as if an egg white was added.

Pineapple Fizz

1 cup	cubed pineapple	250 mL
2 tsp	freshly squeezed lime juice	10 mL
1½ tsp	confectioner's (icing) sugar	7 mL
2 oz	white or amber rum	50 mL
2	ice cubes	2
2 tbsp	soda water or seltzer (approx.)	25 mL

1. In blender, on high speed, blend pineapple, lime juice, sugar, rum and ice until smooth. Pour into a highball glass and top with soda.

Brandy Fizz

1	egg white (or 2 tbsp/25 mL pasteurized liquid egg white)	1
2 tbsp	freshly squeezed lemon juice	25 mL
2 tsp	confectioner's (icing) sugar	10 mL
2 oz	brandy	50 mL
2	ice cubes	2
2 tbsp	soda water or seltzer (approx.)	25 mL

1. In blender, on high speed, blend egg white, lemon juice, sugar, brandy and ice until smooth and frothy. Pour into a highball glass and top with soda.

Citrus Rum Fizz

1	egg white (or 2 tbsp/25 mL pasteurized liquid egg white)	1
¼ cup	orange juice	50 mL
2 tbsp	freshly squeezed lime juice	25 mL
1 tbsp	freshly squeezed lemon juice	15 mL
1½ tsp	confectioner's (icing) sugar	7 mL
2 oz	amber rum	50 mL
2	ice cubes	2
2 tbsp	soda water or seltzer (approx.)	25 mL

1. In blender, on high speed, blend egg white, orange, lime and lemon juices, sugar, rum and ice until smooth. Pour into a highball glass and top with soda.

Morning Glory Fizz

1	egg white (or 2 tbsp/25 mL pasteurized liquid egg white)	1
2 tbsp	freshly squeezed lime juice	25 mL
1½ tsp	confectioner's (icing) sugar	7 mL
2 oz	vodka	50 mL
½ oz	anise liqueur, such as Pernod	15 mL
2	ice cubes	2
2 tbsp	soda water or seltzer (approx.)	25 mL

1. In blender, on high speed, blend egg white, lime juice, sugar, vodka, Pernod and ice until smooth. Pour into a highball glass and top with soda.

Sapphire Fizz

1	egg white (or 2 tbsp/25 mL pasteurized liquid egg white)	1
2 tbsp	freshly squeezed lemon juice	25 mL
1 tsp	confectioner's (icing) sugar	5 mL
2 oz	blue curaçao	50 mL
1 oz	gin	25 mL
2	ice cubes	2
3 tbsp	tonic water or soda water	45 mL
1	slice lemon	1

1. In blender, on high speed, blend egg white, lemon juice, sugar, blue curaçao, gin and ice until smooth. Pour into a highball glass and top with tonic water. Garnish with lemon slice.

Blue Lagoon

2 tbsp	freshly squeezed lime juice	25 mL
2 tbsp	Simple Syrup (see recipe, page 237)	25 mL
1 oz	blue curaçao	25 mL
1 oz	gin	25 mL
1 oz	vodka	25 mL
2	ice cubes	2

1. In blender, on high speed, blend lime juice, Simple Syrup, blue curaçao, gin, vodka and ice until ice is well crushed. Pour into an old-fashioned glass.

Arctic Sunrise

¼ cup	frozen orange juice concentrate	50 mL
2 oz	tequila	50 mL
6	ice cubes	6
1½ tsp	grenadine	7 mL
1	slice orange	1

1. In blender, on high speed, blend orange juice concentrate, tequila and ice until smooth. Pour into a highball glass and top with grenadine. Garnish with orange slice.

You might be tempted to try this drink with breakfast, but I recommend it as an aperitif, despite its name.

Rosy Sunrise

1	orange or tangerine, peeled and seeded	1
1 tsp	grenadine	5 mL
1½ oz	tequila	40 mL

1. In blender, on high speed, blend orange, grenadine and tequila until smooth. Pour into an old-fashioned glass, over ice, if desired.

Salty Star Surprise

1	large star fruit	1
1 tbsp	freshly squeezed lime juice	15 mL
¼ tsp	salt	1 mL
2 oz	tequila or vodka	50 mL
3	ice cubes	3

1. Cut off waxy ridge of each section of star fruit. Cut off sections, discarding core and seeds.

2. In blender, on high speed, blend star fruit, lime juice, salt, tequila and ice until slushy. Pour into an old-fashioned glass.

Bampira on the Roof

¼ cup	pomegranate seeds (or 2 tbsp/25 mL pomegranate juice)	50 mL
2 tbsp	orange juice	25 mL
1 tbsp	freshly squeezed lime juice	15 mL
Pinch	freshly ground black pepper	Pinch
Dash	hot pepper sauce	Dash
2 oz	tequila	50 mL
	Coarse salt, for rimming	

1. In blender, on high speed, blend pomegranate seeds, orange juice, lime juice, pepper, hot pepper sauce and tequila until flesh from pomegranate separates from seed cores. Strain through a fine sieve into an old-fashioned glass rimmed with salt and filled with ice.

Frozen Margarita

2	ice cubes	2
1 tbsp	freshly squeezed lime juice	15 mL
2 oz	tequila	50 mL
1/2 oz	orange liqueur	1 mL
	Coarse salt, for rimming	

1. In blender, pulse ice cubes until crushed. On high speed, blend in lime juice, tequila and orange liqueur until slushy. Serve in a margarita glass rimmed with salt.

Frozen Strawberry Margarita

1	ice cube	1
10	frozen strawberries	10
2 tbsp	strawberry syrup	25 mL
1 tbsp	freshly squeezed lime juice	15 mL
2 tsp	freshly squeezed lemon juice	10 mL
2 oz	tequila	50 mL
1/2 oz	orange liqueur	15 mL
	Coarse salt, for rimming	

1. In blender, pulse ice and strawberries until ice is crushed. On high speed, blend in strawberry syrup, lime and lemon juices, tequila and orange liqueur until slushy. Serve in a margarita glass rimmed with salt.

Frozen Peach Margarita

2	ice cubes	2
½ cup	cubed peeled peaches (see tip, page 244)	125 mL
2 tbsp	freshly squeezed lime juice	25 mL
½ tsp	confectioner's (icing) sugar	2 mL
1 oz	tequila	25 mL
1 oz	orange liqueur	25 mL
1 oz	peach schnapps	25 mL
	Coarse salt, for rimming	

1. In blender, pulse ice and peach until ice is crushed. On high speed, blend in lime juice, sugar, tequila, orange liqueur and peach schnapps until slushy. Serve in a margarita glass rimmed with salt.

Blender Bellini

2	ice cubes	2
½ cup	cubed peeled peaches (see tip, page 244)	125 mL
2 tsp	freshly squeezed lemon juice	10 mL
1 tsp	grenadine	5 mL
½ oz	peach schnapps	15 mL
2 oz	chilled sparkling wine	50 mL

1. In blender, pulse ice and peach until ice is crushed. On high speed, blend in lemon juice, grenadine and peach schnapps until slushy. Pour into a wide-mouthed champagne glass or a martini glass and top with sparkling wine.

Sour Cherry Jubilee

1/4 cup	orange juice	50 mL
1/4 cup	drained jarred sour cherries	50 mL
2 oz	rye whisky	50 mL
2 dashes	angostura bitters	2 dashes
2	ice cubes	2
1	maraschino cherry	1

1. In blender, on high speed, blend orange juice, cherries, whisky, bitters and ice until smooth. Pour into an old-fashioned glass and garnish with maraschino cherry.

Peaches 'n' Cream

1/2 cup	cubed peeled peaches (see tip, page 244)	125 mL
1/2 cup	half-and-half (10%) cream	125 mL
1 oz	brandy	25 mL
1 oz	peach schnapps	25 mL
2	ice cubes	2

1. In blender, on high speed, blend peach, cream, brandy, peach schnapps and ice until smooth. Pour into an old-fashioned glass.

Freezing Navel

1/4 cup	frozen orange juice concentrate	50 mL
2 oz	peach schnapps	50 mL
6	ice cubes	6
1	slice peach or orange	1

1. In blender, on high speed, blend orange juice concentrate, peach schnapps and ice until slushy. Pour into a highball glass and garnish with peach slice.

Peach Sparkler

½ cup	cubed peeled peaches (see tip, page 244)	125 mL
1 oz	peach schnapps	25 mL
2	ice cubes	2
2 oz	chilled sparkling wine	50 mL

1. In blender, on high speed, blend peaches, peach schnapps and ice until smooth. Pour into a wine glass and top with sparkling wine.

Raspberry Peach Sparkler

⅓ cup	cubed peeled peaches (see tip, page 244)	75 mL
⅓ cup	fresh or frozen raspberries	75 mL
1 oz	peach schnapps	25 mL
6	ice cubes	6
2 oz	chilled sparkling wine	50 mL

1. In blender, on high speed, blend peaches, raspberries, peach schnapps and ice until slushy. Pour into a large wine glass and top with sparkling wine.

Blueberry Sparkler

¼ cup	blueberries	50 mL
1 oz	blue curaçao	25 mL
3 oz	chilled sparkling wine	75 mL

1. In blender, on high speed, blend all but 3 of the blueberries and blue curaçao until berries are well crushed. Strain through a fine sieve into a flute and top with sparkling wine. Garnish with reserved berries.

Pineapple Sparkler

½ cup	cubed pineapple	125 mL
1 tbsp	freshly squeezed lime juice	15 mL
½ oz	amber rum	15 mL
2	ice cubes	2
3 oz	chilled sparkling wine	75 mL

1. In blender, on high speed, blend pineapple, lime juice, rum and ice until smooth. Pour into a large wine glass and top with sparkling wine.

Mango Sparkler

½ cup	cubed peeled mango	125 mL
2 tbsp	orange juice	25 mL
½ oz	brandy	15 mL
2	ice cubes	2
2 oz	chilled sparkling wine	50 mL

1. In blender, on high speed, blend mango, orange juice, brandy and ice until smooth. Pour into a wine glass and top with sparkling wine.

Persimmon Sparkler

½ cup	cubed peeled very ripe persimmon	125 mL
2 tbsp	orange juice	25 mL
½ oz	brandy	15 mL
2	ice cubes	2
2 oz	chilled sparkling wine	50 mL

1. In blender, on high speed, blend persimmon, orange juice, brandy and ice until smooth. Pour into a wine glass and top with sparkling wine.

Maple Leaf

1 tbsp	freshly squeezed lemon juice	15 mL
1 tbsp	pure maple syrup	15 mL
2 oz	rye whisky	50 mL
2	ice cubes	2

1. In blender, on high speed, blend lemon juice, maple syrup, whisky and ice until slushy. Pour into an old-fashioned glass.

Mary's Milkshake

⅓ cup	vanilla ice cream	75 mL
2 tbsp	milk	25 mL
2 oz	brandy	50 mL
¾ oz	crème de cacao	22 mL

1. In blender, on high speed, blend ice cream, milk and brandy until smooth. Pour into an old-fashioned glass and drizzle with crème de cacao.

Strawberry Shake

6	fresh or frozen strawberries	6
¼ cup	vanilla ice cream	50 mL
2 oz	white or amber rum	50 mL
½ oz	orange liqueur	15 mL
1	fresh strawberry (optional)	1

1. In blender, on high speed, blend strawberries, ice cream, rum and orange liqueur until smooth. Pour into an old-fashioned glass and garnish with strawberry, if desired.

Madeira M'Dear

6	fresh or frozen strawberries	6
1/4 cup	vanilla ice cream	50 mL
2 oz	Madeira	25 mL
1	fresh strawberry (optional)	1

1. In blender, on high speed, blend strawberries, ice cream and Madeira until smooth. Pour into an old-fashioned glass and garnish with strawberry, if desired.

This traditional drink is for those who cannot decide if they want a post-prandial ice cream or a drink.

White Cargo

| 1/4 cup | vanilla ice cream | 50 mL |
| 2 oz | gin | 50 mL |

1. In blender, on high speed, blend ice cream and gin until smooth. Pour into an old-fashioned glass.

Peach Almond Shake

1/2 cup	cubed peeled peaches (see tip, page 244)	125 mL
1/3 cup	vanilla ice cream	75 mL
2 tsp	freshly squeezed lemon juice	10 mL
1 oz	brandy	25 mL
1 oz	peach schnapps	25 mL
1 oz	almond liqueur	25 mL
1	ice cube	1

1. In blender, on high speed, blend peach, ice cream, lemon juice, brandy, peach schnapps, almond liqueur and ice until smooth. Pour into an old-fashioned glass.

MAKES 1 SERVING

For a lower-alcohol version, reduce the vodka and increase the milk by equal amounts.

White Russian Shake

1/3 cup	vanilla ice cream	75 mL
2 tbsp	milk	25 mL
3 oz	vodka	45 mL
1 oz	coffee liqueur, such as Kahlúa	15 mL

1. In blender, on high speed, blend ice cream, milk, vodka and coffee liqueur until smooth. Pour into an old-fashioned glass.

MAKES 1 SERVING

For a lower-alcohol version, reduce the vodka and increase the milk by equal amounts.

Brown Russian Shake

1/4 cup	chocolate ice cream	50 mL
2 tbsp	milk	25 mL
3 oz	vodka	75 mL
1 1/2 oz	coffee liqueur, such as Kahlúa	40 mL
2	ice cubes	2
2 tsp	grated bittersweet chocolate	10 mL

1. In blender, on high speed, blend ice cream, milk, vodka, coffee liqueur and ice until smooth. Pour into an old-fashioned glass and sprinkle with chocolate.

MAKES 1 SERVING

Frozen Mudslide

1/2 cup	vanilla ice cream	125 mL
1/2 cup	milk	125 mL
2 oz	Irish cream liqueur	50 mL
1 oz	coffee liqueur, such as Kahlúa	25 mL
1 oz	vodka	25 mL
1	ice cube	1
1 tbsp	grated bittersweet chocolate	15 mL

1. In blender, on high speed, blend ice cream, milk, Irish cream liqueur, coffee liqueur, vodka and ice until smooth. Pour into an old-fashioned glass and sprinkle with chocolate.

Truffle in a Glass

¼ cup	chocolate ice cream	50 mL
1 oz	hazelnut liqueur	25 mL
4	ice cubes	4
1 tsp	grated bittersweet chocolate (optional)	5 mL

1. In blender, on high speed, blend ice cream, hazelnut liqueur and ice until smooth. Pour into an old-fashioned glass and sprinkle with chocolate, if desired.

Mint Truffle Shake

¼ cup	chocolate ice cream	50 mL
1 oz	hazelnut liqueur	25 mL
½ oz	white crème de menthe	15 mL
4	ice cubes	4
1 tsp	grated bittersweet chocolate (optional)	5 mL

1. In blender, on high speed, blend ice cream, hazelnut liqueur, crème de menthe and ice until smooth. Pour into an old-fashioned glass and sprinkle with chocolate, if desired.

Irish Cream Coffee

¼ cup	cold brewed espresso coffee	50 mL
¼ cup	chocolate ice cream	50 mL
3 oz	Irish cream liqueur	75 mL

1. In blender, on high speed, blend coffee, ice cream and Irish cream liqueur until smooth. Pour into an old-fashioned glass or a coffee cup.

Banana Splish-Splash

1	banana	1
½ cup	cubed pineapple	125 mL
¼ cup	orange juice	50 mL
¼ cup	vanilla ice cream	50 mL
1 ½ oz	amber or dark rum	40 mL
½ oz	coconut rum	15 mL
3	ice cubes	3

1. In blender, on high speed, blend banana, pineapple, orange juice, ice cream, amber and coconut rums and ice until slushy. Pour into a milkshake glass or a tall stemmed punch glass.

MAKES 1 SERVING

Mint Jubilee

¼ cup	vanilla ice cream	50 mL
2 oz	bourbon	50 mL
1 oz	white crème de menthe	25 mL
1	fresh mint leaf (optional)	1

1. In blender, on high speed, blend ice cream, bourbon and crème de menthe until smooth. Pour into an old-fashioned glass and garnish with mint, if desired.

MAKES 1 SERVING

This fabulous dessert drink features the classic French combination of Armagnac and prunes (the equivalent of North America's rum and raisin).

The Capital "S"

¼ cup	vanilla ice cream	50 mL
2	pitted prunes	2
2 oz	Armagnac	50 mL

1. In blender, on high speed, blend ice cream, prunes and Armagnac until prunes are very finely chopped but not puréed. Pour into an old-fashioned glass.

Jack Splat

¼ cup	caramel ice cream	50 mL
2 oz	Tennessee whiskey	50 mL
1	ice cube	1
½ tsp	liquid honey	2 mL
	Dark brown sugar, for rimming	
1 tsp	whipping (35%) cream	5 mL

1. In blender, on high speed, blend ice cream, whiskey and ice until smooth. Wet the rim of an old-fashioned glass with honey and dip in sugar. Pour ice cream mixture into glass and drizzle with whipping cream.

Raspberry Freezie

¼ cup	raspberry sorbet	50 mL
2 oz	chilled framboise	50 mL
2 tsp	grated bittersweet chocolate	10 mL
	Fresh raspberries, for garnish	

1. In blender, on high speed, blend sorbet and framboise until smooth. Pour into a martini glass, sprinkle with chocolate and garnish with raspberries.

Filipino Avocado Dream

½	avocado, peeled	½
2 tbsp	sweetened condensed milk	25 mL
2 oz	white or amber rum	50 mL
3	ice cubes	3

1. In blender, on high speed, blend avocado, condensed milk, rum and ice until smooth. Pour into an old-fashioned glass.

For a petite after-dinner treat for 4, serve in small chocolate cups.

Polar Express

¼ cup	brewed espresso coffee, cooled	50 mL
2 tbsp	sweetened condensed milk	25 mL
1 oz	brandy	25 mL
½ oz	almond or hazelnut liqueur	15 mL
2	ice cubes	2

1. In blender, on high speed, blend coffee, condensed milk, brandy, almond liqueur and ice until smooth. Pour into an old-fashioned glass.

Frozen B-52

2	ice cubes	2
1 oz	Irish cream liqueur	25 mL
1 oz	orange brandy	25 mL
1 oz	coffee liqueur, such as Kahlúa	25 mL

1. In blender, pulse ice until crushed. On high speed, blend in Irish cream liqueur, orange brandy and coffee liqueur until slushy. Pour into an old-fashioned glass.

Cuban Morning

¼ cup	brewed espresso coffee, cooled	50 mL
1 tbsp	whipping (35%) cream	15 mL
	Confectioner's (icing) sugar	
1½ oz	amber rum (preferably aged Cuban rum)	40 mL
2	ice cubes	2

1. In blender, on high speed, blend coffee, whipping cream, sugar to taste, rum and ice until smooth. Pour into an old-fashioned glass or a coffee cup.

This is a nutritious, cleansing hangover drink. For a non-bitter drink, substitute peeled and seeded cucumber for the bitter melon.

This recipe contains a raw egg. If the food safety of raw eggs is a concern for you, use the pasteurized liquid whole egg instead.

Bitter Morning

1	egg (or ¼ cup/50 mL pasteurized liquid whole egg)	1
1 cup	chopped seeded bitter melon	250 mL
Pinch	salt	Pinch
Pinch	freshly ground black pepper	Pinch
Dash	Worcestershire sauce	Dash
Dash	hot pepper sauce	Dash
2 oz	vodka	50 mL
3	ice cubes	3

1. In blender, on high speed, blend egg, bitter melon, salt, pepper, Worcestershire sauce, hot pepper sauce, vodka and ice until smooth. Pour into a highball glass.

Cherries are known for their gout-preventive properties. But everyone will enjoy this cocktail, not just those who suffer from gout.

Gout Potion

¼ cup	drained canned sweet or sour cherries	50 mL
¼ cup	sweet or sour cherry juice or cranberry cocktail	50 mL
2 oz	vodka	50 mL
4	ice cubes	4

1. In blender, on high speed, blend cherries, cherry juice, vodka and ice until smooth. Pour into an old-fashioned glass.

Although there are no true hangover remedies, this might make you feel better for a while — and you get a little nutrition at the same time.

Hair of the Clam

1	peeled very ripe tomato or canned tomato	1
2 tbsp	clam juice	25 mL
2½ tsp	freshly squeezed lemon juice, divided	12 mL
Pinch	salt	Pinch
Pinch	freshly ground black pepper	Pinch
Dash	hot pepper sauce	Dash
2 oz	vodka or aquavit	50 mL
1	ice cube	1
	Celery salt, for rimming	
1	short stalk celery	1

1. In blender, on high speed, blend tomato, clam juice, 2 tsp (10 mL) of the lemon juice, salt, pepper, hot pepper sauce, vodka and ice until smooth. Wet the rim of an old-fashioned glass with the remaining ½ tsp (2 mL) lemon juice and dip in celery salt. Pour drink into glass and garnish with celery stalk.

Baby Food

EIGHT MONTHS AND OLDER

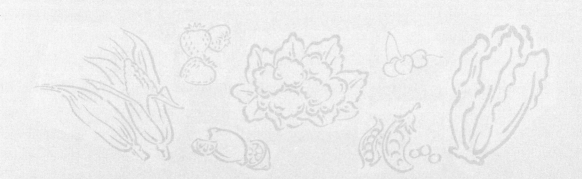

NINE MONTHS AND OLDER

TWELVE MONTHS AND OLDER

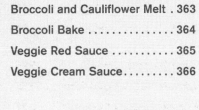

Introduction to Baby Food

Baby food doesn't have to come in jars. Making your own at home is not difficult. Baby food is simply strained, puréed or mashed adult food, just a different version of the food you prepare for yourself. Here are three good reasons to make your own baby food:

- You know what's in it.
- You can tailor the texture to your baby's preferences.
- You can shape your baby's tastes and help her learn what fresh foods taste like.

Whether you choose to make all your own baby food, or just some of it, the blender is a great way to offer new flavors in a baby-friendly texture. Even when your child is eating table food, you can always find an occasion for a fruit smoothie or a nutritious blended dip.

Most babies start eating solid foods between 4 and 6 months. At this point, they are both mentally and physiologically ready to accept solid foods. Every baby is different when it comes to their readiness to start solid foods.

The recipes that follow are accompanied by an age guideline. Remember, these are just suggestions. Your pediatrician or family doctor may suggest otherwise, especially if you have a family history of allergies or intolerances. When it comes to textures and flavors, let your baby guide you. He will let you know when he is ready for something new. Here's a general idea of what foods are safe when:

4–6 months:	Single vegetables and fruits (after you've started with single-grain cereal)
> 6 months:	Mixed vegetables and fruits (after all ingredients in the recipe have been introduced separately, which helps to identify allergies or intolerances)
> 7 months:	Pasta, rice, other grains
> 8 months:	Meat, chicken, fish, lentils, egg yolks
> 9 months:	Yogurt, cheese
> 12 months:	Homogenized milk, honey and all potentially allergenic foods (nuts and nut butters, egg whites)

TIPS FOR MAKING BABY FOOD

- Work under the most sanitary conditions possible:
  - Scrub your hands with hot water and soap, rinse and dry with clean towel before fixing your baby's food, before feeding your baby and after changing your baby's diapers.
  - Scrub all working surfaces with soap and hot water.
  - Scrub all equipment with soap and hot water, and rinse well.
- Prepare fresh fruits and vegetables by scrubbing, paring or peeling and removing seeds.
- Prepare meats by removing all bones, skin, connective tissue, gristle and fat.
- Cook foods, when necessary, by boiling them in a small, covered saucepan with a small amount of water until tender. The amount of water is important: the less water used, the more nutrients stay in the food.
- Purée food using a blender, food processor, baby food grinder, spoon or fork. Grind up tough foods. Cut food into small pieces or thin slices. Remove seeds and pits from fruit.
- *There's no need to add salt or sugar.*
- Avoid deep-frying, which adds unhealthy fats to foods.
- Don't feel you have to prepare separate meals for your baby. You can simply take portions of your adult food (before you add salt) and grind or mash it to a consistency appropriate for your baby.
- Make enough purée for several meals and store as directed below or in the recipe.

TO STORE

- If you're not using puréed food right away, refrigerate or freeze it in portioned containers. Most refrigerated foods will last up to 3 days (exceptions are noted in the recipes).
- To freeze: Pour cooled, puréed food into a clean ice cube tray and cover with plastic wrap or foil. When frozen solid (after about 24 hours), transfer cubes to a resealable freezer bag labeled with the contents and date.
- Rotate stock as the supermarket does, putting the most recently frozen foods behind the previously frozen ones.

TO THAW/REHEAT

- For slow thawing, place a day's worth of baby food in a sealed container in the refrigerator. It will thaw in about 4 hours. Do not thaw at room temperature, as bacteria could grow in the food while it is thawing.
- For fast thawing and heating, heat frozen cubes in a heat-resistant container in a pan of hot water over low heat or in the microwave.
- Stir the food well and test it with a finger to be sure it's not too hot (especially if you use a microwave). Babies generally like their food close to room temperature.
- Discard any food that has been heated and not eaten.

— Nicole Young

**MAKES ABOUT
2 CUPS (500 ML)**

Apples are a good source of soluble fiber, which helps with bowel function and may lower cholesterol levels.

Apples

| 4 cups | chopped peeled apples (about 4) | 1 L |
| ½ cup | water | 125 mL |

1. In a medium saucepan, over medium-low heat, bring apples and water to a simmer, covered, stirring occasionally, until apples are very tender, about 20 minutes.

2. Transfer apples to blender and purée on high speed.

Nutritional Information (Per ¼-cup/50 mL Serving)

Calories: 12 Kcal; Total Carbohydrates: 3 g; Fibre: 1 g; Fat: 0 g; Protein: 0 g; Iron: 0 mg

---

**MAKES ABOUT
2 CUPS (500 ML)**

Apricots

| 2 cups | apricots | 500 mL |
| ¼ cup | water | 50 mL |

1. In a small saucepan of boiling water, blanch apricots for 30 seconds. Remove stones from apricots and chop.

2. Place in blender with ¼ cup (50 mL) water and purée on high speed.

Nutritional Information (Per ¼-cup/50 mL Serving)

Calories: 18 Kcal; Total Carbohydrates: 4 g; Fiber: 1 g; Fat: 0 g; Protein: 0 g; Iron: 0 mg

---

**MAKES ABOUT
½ CUP (125 ML)**

This "peel and mash" fruit is always quick, convenient and nutritious. Bananas are high in potassium and vitamin B6.

TIP

Freeze chunks of unblemished bananas on a baking sheet in a single layer. When frozen, transfer to a resealable bag and freeze for up to 6 months.

Banana

1	very ripe banana	1

1. In blender, on high speed, purée banana.
2. *Make ahead:* Store in an airtight container in the refrigerator for up to 1 day.

Nutritional Information (Per ¼-cup/50 mL Serving)

Calories: 80 Kcal; Total Carbohydrates: 20 g; Fiber: 2 g; Fat: 0 g; Protein: 1 g; Iron: 0 mg

---

**MAKES ABOUT
2 CUPS (500 ML)**

Blueberries are fine to purée on high speed without cooking, but tend to be more tart that way.

TIP

Make up a batch of this recipe and blend a frozen cube of it (see introduction, page 285) with any fruit favorite, such as apples, pears or bananas.

Blueberries

2 cups	blueberries (about 12 oz/375 g)	500 mL
½ cup	water	125 mL

1. In a medium saucepan, over medium heat, bring blueberries and water just to a boil. Cover, reduce heat and simmer for 15 minutes, until berries are very tender. Let cool.
2. Transfer blueberries to blender and purée on high speed.
3. Push through a fine sieve with a wooden spoon to remove any seeds that may be offensive to your baby.

Nutritional Information (Per ¼-cup/50 mL Serving)

Calories: 20 Kcal; Total Carbohydrates: 5 g; Fiber: 1 g; Fat: 0 g; Protein: 0 g; Iron: 0 mg

MAKES 2 CUPS (500 ML)

Summer sweet cherries are the ultimate treat!

TIP

Cherries can be purchased already pitted and chilled, and can be portioned out and frozen to enjoy all year long.

Cherries

| 2 cups | pitted sweet red or black cherries (about 1 lb/500 g) | 500 mL |

1. In blender, on high speed, purée cherries.

> **Nutritional Information (Per ¼-cup/50 mL Serving)**
>
> Calories: 18 Kcal; Total Carbohydrates: 4 g; Fiber: 1 g; Fat: 0 g; Protein: 0 g; Iron: 0 mg

MAKES ABOUT 2 CUPS (500 ML)

Fresh figs are a good source of potassium and fiber; they also tend to have laxative properties.

TIP

If your baby is texture-sensitive, push the purée through a fine sieve with a wooden spoon to get a very smooth consistency.

Figs

| 2 cups | black figs, stems removed (about 8 oz/227 g) | 500 mL |
| ½ cup | water | 125 mL |

1. In a medium saucepan, over medium heat, bring figs and water just to a boil. Cover, reduce heat and simmer until figs are very tender, about 15 minutes. Let cool.

2. Transfer figs to blender and purée on high speed.

> **Nutritional Information (Per ¼-cup/50 mL Serving)**
>
> Calories: 37 Kcal; Total Carbohydrates: 10 g; Fiber: 2 g; Fat: 0 g; Protein: 0 g; Iron: 0 mg

Kiwi

**MAKES ABOUT
2 CUPS (500 ML)**

*Kiwis are high in
vitamins C and E and
act as antioxidants.
They have a rich,
buttery texture that
appeals to babies.*

TIP

Choose kiwis that
are firm but yield to
gentle pressure. Place
them in a brown
paper bag to ripen.

3 cups	chopped peeled kiwis (about 6)	750 mL

1. In blender, on high speed, purée kiwis.
2. *Make ahead:* Store in the refrigerator for up to 3 days.
   Do not freeze.

> **Nutritional Information (Per ¼-cup/50 mL Serving)**
>
> Calories: 27 Kcal; Total Carbohydrates: 7 g; Fiber: 1 g;
> Fat: 0 g; Protein: 0 g; Iron: 0 mg; Vitamin C: 43 mg

Mango

**MAKES ABOUT
2 CUPS (500 ML)**

*Mangoes help the
body maintain bowel
regularity and fight
infection. The skin
can irritate a baby's
mouth, so always peel
before using.*

TIP

Mangoes should have
unblemished red and
yellow skin that yields
slightly to pressure. If
mango is very fibrous,
push puréed mango
through a fine sieve
with a wooden spoon
to give a smooth
creamy consistency.

3 cups	chopped peeled mangoes (about 2 large)	750 mL
¼ cup	water	50 mL

1. In blender, on high speed, purée mangoes and water.

> **Nutritional Information (Per ¼-cup/50 mL Serving)**
>
> Calories: 27 Kcal; Total Carbohydrates: 7 g; Fiber: 1 g;
> Fat: 0 g; Protein: 0 g; Iron: 0 mg

Melon

| 3 cups | cubed cantaloupe or honeydew melon (about $\frac{1}{2}$) | 750 mL |

1. In blender, on high speed, purée melon.

Nutritional Information (Per $\frac{1}{4}$-cup/50 mL Serving)

Calories: 5 Kcal; Total Carbohydrates: 1 g; Fiber: 0 g;
Fat: 0 g; Protein: 0 g; Iron: 0 mg

Nectarines

**MAKES ABOUT
2 CUPS (500 ML)**

| 3 cups | chopped nectarines (about 4) | 750 mL |
| $\frac{1}{4}$ cup | water | 50 mL |

1. In blender, on high speed, purée nectarines and water.

Nutritional Information (Per $\frac{1}{4}$-cup/50 mL Serving)

Calories: 17 Kcal; Total Carbohydrates: 4 g; Fiber: 1 g;
Fat: 0 g; Protein: 0 g; Iron: 0 mg

Papaya

**MAKES ABOUT
2 CUPS (500 ML)**

*Papaya is an excellent
source of vitamin C
and a good source
of potassium and
vitamin A.*

TIP

Avoid papayas that are
hard and green: they
will never ripen.

| 3 cups | chopped peeled papaya (about 2) | 750 mL |
| $\frac{1}{4}$ cup | water | 50 mL |

1. In blender, on high speed, purée papaya and water.

Nutritional Information (Per $\frac{1}{4}$-cup/50 mL Serving)

Calories: 20 Kcal; Total Carbohydrates: 5 g; Fiber: 1 g;
Fat: 0 g; Protein: 0 g; Iron: 0 mg; Vitamin C: 32 mg

**MAKES ABOUT
2 CUPS (500 ML)**

TIP

Substitute 3 cups
(750 mL) frozen
unsweetened sliced
peaches if fresh are
not available.

Peaches

| 4 | peaches | 4 |
| 1/2 cup | water | 125 mL |

1. In a small saucepan of boiling water, blanch peaches for 30 seconds. Plunge into cold water. Remove peel and stones from peaches and chop to make about 3 cups (750 mL).

2. Place in blender, add water and purée on high speed.

Nutritional Information (Per 1/4-cup/50 mL Serving)
Calories: 18 Kcal; Total Carbohydrates: 5 g; Fiber: 1 g; Fat: 0 g; Iron: 0 mg; Protein: 0 g

**MAKES ABOUT
2 CUPS (500 ML)**

*Pears are a sweet
source of soluble fiber.*

TIP

Very ripe pears can be
washed, peeled, cored,
chopped and puréed
without cooking.

Pears

| 3 cups | chopped peeled pears (about 4) | 750 mL |
| 1/2 cup | water | 125 mL |

1. In a medium saucepan, over medium-low heat, bring pears and water to a simmer, covered, stirring occasionally, until pears are very tender, about 20 minutes. Let cool.

2. Transfer pears to blender and purée on high speed.

Nutritional Information (Per 1/4-cup/50 mL Serving)
Calories: 24 Kcal; Total Carbohydrates: 6 g; Fiber: 1 g; Fat: 0 g; Protein: 0 g; Iron: 0 mg

**MAKES ABOUT
2 CUPS (500 ML)**

Plums

| 3 cups | chopped plums (about 6) | 750 mL |
| 1/2 cup | water | 125 mL |

1. In a medium saucepan, over medium-low heat, bring plums and water to a simmer, covered, stirring occasionally, until plums are very tender, about 20 minutes. Let cool.

2. Transfer plums to blender and purée on high speed.

Nutritional Information (Per 1/4-cup/50 mL Serving)

Calories: 23 Kcal; Total Carbohydrates: 5 g; Fiber: 1 g; Fat: 0 g; Protein: 0 g; Iron: 0 mg

---

**MAKES ABOUT
2 CUPS (500 ML)**

These natural laxatives should be used in moderation unless constipation is an issue.

TIP

If your baby is texture-sensitive, push the purée through a fine sieve with a wooden spoon to get a very smooth consistency.

Prunes

| 1 1/2 cups | pitted prunes (about 8 oz/250 g) | 375 mL |
| 1/2 cup | water | 125 mL |

1. In a medium saucepan, over medium heat, bring prunes and water just to a boil. Cover, reduce heat and simmer until prunes are very tender, about 15 minutes. Let cool.

2. Transfer prunes to blender and purée on high speed.

Nutritional Information (Per 1/4-cup/50 mL Serving)

Calories: 75 Kcal; Total Carbohydrates: 20 g; Fiber: 2 g; Fat: 0 g; Protein: 1 g; Iron: 0 mg

**MAKES ABOUT
2 CUPS (500 ML)**

Berries are sometimes hard on little tummies. Try berries when baby has tried many of the other fruits and vegetables and the digestive tract is more developed. Make sure to watch for a reaction.

TIP

Use an equal amount of frozen berries when fresh are not in season.

Strawberries, Raspberries and Blackberries

| 2 cups | fresh raspberries, blackberries or sliced strawberries | 500 mL |
| ½ cup | water | 125 mL |

1. In blender, on high speed, purée berries and water.
2. Push through a fine sieve with a wooden spoon to remove any seeds.

Nutritional Information (Per ¼-cup/50 mL Serving)

Raspberries
Calories: 16 Kcal; Total Carbohydrates: 4 g; Fiber: 2 g;
Fat: 0 g; Protein: 0 g; Iron: 0 mg
Blackberries
Calories: 19 Kcal; Total Carbohydrates: 5 g; Fiber: 2 g;
Fat: 0 g; Protein: 0 g; Iron: 0 mg
Strawberries
Calories: 11 Kcal; Total Carbohydrates: 3 g; Fiber: 1 g;
Fat: 0 g; Protein: 0 g; Iron: 0 mg; Vitamin C: 21 mg

**MAKES ABOUT
2 CUPS (500 ML)**

The high water content of melons makes them very refreshing for little palates.

TIP

Choose melons that are fragrant and heavy for their size.

Watermelon

| 2½ cups | chopped seedless watermelon | 375 mL |

1. In blender, on high speed, purée watermelon.

Nutritional Information (Per ¼-cup/50 mL Serving)

Calories: 15 Kcal; Total Carbohydrates: 3 g; Fiber: 0 g;
Fat: 0 g; Protein: 0 g; Iron: 0 mg

Avocado

| ¼ cup | chopped peeled avocado (about ½) | 50 mL |

1. In blender, on high speed, purée avocado.

Nutritional Information (Per ¼-cup/50 mL Serving)

Calories: 59 Kcal; Total Carbohydrates: 3 g; Fiber: 1 g;
Fat: 6 g; Protein: 1 g; Iron: 0 mg

Beets

| 2 cups | chopped peeled beets (about 1 bunch) | 500 mL |
| ½ cup | water | 125 mL |

1. In a medium saucepan, over medium heat, bring beets
   and water just to a boil. Cover, reduce heat and simmer
   until very tender, about 20 minutes. Let cool.
2. Transfer beets to blender and purée on high speed.

Nutritional Information (Per ¼-cup/50 mL Serving)

Calories: 15 Kcal; Total Carbohydrates: 1 g; Fiber: 1 g;
Fat: 0 g; Protein: 1 g; Iron: 0 mg

Broccoli Stems and Florets

MAKES ABOUT
2 CUPS (500 ML)

Cooked broccoli is an excellent source of vitamin C and potassium.

TIPS

Use a vegetable peeler to remove the fibrous skin from broccoli stems.

Once your baby is used to the flavor of broccoli, use the same cooking method with 2½ cups (625 mL) florets (the texture of the buds can be off-putting to younger children).

1½ cups	sliced peeled broccoli stems (see tips, at left)	375 mL
1 cup	water	250 mL

1. In a medium saucepan, over medium heat, bring stems and water to a boil. Cover, reduce heat and simmer until broccoli is very tender, about 15 minutes. Let cool.

2. Transfer broccoli to blender and purée on high speed.

> **Nutritional Information (Per ¼-cup/50 mL Serving)**
>
> Calories: 8 Kcal; Total Carbohydrates: 1 g; Fiber: 0 g; Fat: 0 g; Protein: 1 g; Iron: 0 mg; Vitamin C: 26 mg

Cabbage

MAKES ABOUT
2 CUPS (500 ML)

Green, red, Savoy, Napa and bok choy are some of the different varieties of this nutrient-dense vegetable. They can all be prepared in the same manner.

3 cups	chopped cabbage (about 8 oz/250 g)	750 mL

1. Place cabbage in a steamer basket fitted over a saucepan of boiling water; cover and steam for 15 to 20 minutes, or until very tender. Let cool.

2. Transfer cabbage to blender and purée on high speed, adding water if necessary.

> **Nutritional Information (Per ¼-cup/50 mL Serving)**
>
> Calories: 8 Kcal; Total Carbohydrates: 2 g; Fiber: 1 g; Fat: 0 g; Protein: 0 g; Iron: 0 mg

**MAKES ABOUT
2 CUPS (500 ML)**

Carrots

| 2 cups | chopped peeled carrots (about 4) | 500 mL |
| 1 cup | water | 125 mL |

1. In a medium saucepan, over medium heat, bring carrots and water just to a boil. Cover, reduce heat and simmer until carrots are very tender, about 15 minutes. Let cool.

2. Transfer carrots to blender and purée on high speed.

Nutritional Information (Per 1/4-cup/50 mL Serving)

Calories: 14 Kcal; Total Carbohydrates: 3 g; Fiber: 1 g; Fat: 0 g; Protein: 0 g; Iron: 0 mg

**MAKES ABOUT
2 CUPS (500 ML)**

Cauliflower is the most easily digestible member of the cabbage family and is a great introduction to the cruciferous group, which also includes cabbage, broccoli, Brussels sprouts, collard greens and kohlrabi.

TIP

Add a piece of bread to the water when boiling to absorb some of the odor. Discard bread before puréeing.

Cauliflower

| 2 1/2 cups | cauliflower florets | 375 mL |
| 1 cup | water | 250 mL |

1. In a medium saucepan, over medium heat, bring cauliflower and water just to a boil. Cover, reduce heat and simmer until cauliflower is very tender, about 10 minutes. Let cool.

2. Transfer cauliflower to blender and purée on high speed.

Nutritional Information (Per 1/4-cup/50 mL Serving)

Calories: 8 Kcal; Total Carbohydrates: 2 g; Fiber: 1 g; Fat: 0 g; Protein: 0 g; Iron: 0 mg

**MAKES 2 CUPS
(500 ML)**

*This is one vegetable
that is easier to use
when frozen.*

Corn

| 2 cups | fresh or frozen corn kernels | 500 mL |
| ½ cup | water | 125 mL |

1. In a medium saucepan, over medium heat, bring corn
and water just to a boil. Cover, reduce heat and simmer
until corn is tender, about 3 minutes. Let cool.

2. Transfer corn to blender and purée on high speed.

Nutritional Information (Per ¼-cup/50 mL Serving)

Calories: 49 Kcal; Total Carbohydrates: 12 g; Fiber: 1 g;
Fat: 0 g; Protein: 2 g; Iron: 0 mg

**MAKES ABOUT
1 CUP (250 ML)**

*Cucumber is very mild
and refreshing. The
waxy skin is not very
palatable for little
ones, so always peel
before using.*

Cucumber

| 1½ cups | cubed peeled and seeded cucumber (about 1 small) | 375 mL |

1. In blender, on high speed, purée cucumber.

2. *Make ahead*: Store in the refrigerator for up to 3 days. Do
not freeze.

Nutritional Information (Per ¼-cup/50 mL Serving)

Calories: 7 Kcal; Total Carbohydrates: 2 g; Fiber: 0 g;
Fat: 0 g; Protein: 0 g; Iron: 0 mg

**MAKES ABOUT
2 CUPS (500 ML)**

Eggplant

- *Preheat oven to 350°F (180°C)*
- *Rimmed baking sheet, lined with foil*

3 cups	cubed peeled eggplant (about 1 small)	750 mL
1 tbsp	olive oil	15 mL
1/4 cup	water	50 mL

1. In a bowl, toss eggplant with oil and spread in a single layer on prepared baking sheet. Bake in preheated oven until eggplant is tender, about 20 minutes. Let cool.
2. Transfer to blender, add water and purée on high speed.

Nutritional Information (Per 1/4-cup/50 mL Serving)

Calories: 8 Kcal; Total Carbohydrates: 2 g; Fiber: 1 g;
Fat: 0 g; Protein: 0 g; Iron: 0 mg

**MAKES ABOUT
2 CUPS (500 ML)**

Green Beans

Choose young green beans that are tender and not too fibrous, and remove any fibers that are on them. French beans make the smoothest purée.

| 3 cups | halved trimmed green beans | 750 mL |
| 2 cups | water | 500 mL |

1. In a large saucepan, over medium-high heat, bring beans and water to a boil. Cover, reduce heat and simmer until beans are very tender, about 15 minutes. Let cool.
2. Transfer beans to blender and purée on high speed.

Nutritional Information (Per 1/4-cup/50 mL Serving)

Calories: 13 Kcal; Total Carbohydrates: 3 g; Fiber: 1 g;
Fat: 0 g; Protein: 1 g; Iron: 0 mg

TIPS

Substitute frozen green beans if fresh are not available.

Push purée through a fine sieve for a smoother consistency.

**MAKES ABOUT
2 CUPS (500 ML)**

*Beet greens, collard
greens, mustard greens,
kale and Swiss chard
all fall into this group,
and all are excellent
sources of vitamin A.*

Dark Leafy Greens

6 cups	chopped dark leafy greens, tough stems and ribs removed	1.5 L
½ cup	water	125 mL

1. Arrange greens in a large nonstick skillet. Pour in water, cover and cook over medium-high heat, stirring occasionally, until greens are very tender, about 15 minutes. Let cool.

2. Transfer greens to blender and purée on high speed, adding water if necessary.

Nutritional Information (Per ¼-cup/50 mL Serving)

Calories: 34 Kcal; Total Carbohydrates: 7 g; Fiber: 1 g; Fat: 0 g; Protein: 2 g; Iron: 1 mg; Vitamin C: 80 mg

**MAKES ABOUT
2 CUPS (500 ML)**

*Cooked okra is an
excellent source of
potassium and is easy
for little ones to digest.*

Okra

2 cups	okra, stems removed	500 mL
1 cup	water	250 mL

1. In a medium saucepan, over medium-high heat, bring okra and water to a boil. Cover, reduce heat and simmer until okra is very tender, about 20 minutes. Let cool.

2. Transfer okra to blender and purée on high speed.

Nutritional Information (Per ¼-cup/50 mL Serving)

Calories: 10 Kcal; Total Carbohydrates: 2 g; Fiber: 1 g; Fat: 0 g; Protein: 1 g; Iron: 0 mg

*Like many other root
vegetables, parsnips
have a mild, sweet
flavor that infants love.*

Parsnips

2 cups	chopped peeled parsnips (about 4)	500 mL
1 cup	water	250 mL

1. In a medium saucepan, over medium heat, bring parsnips and water just to a boil. Cover, reduce heat and simmer until very tender, about 20 minutes. Let cool.

2. Transfer parsnips to blender and purée on high speed.

Nutritional Information (Per ¼-cup/50 mL Serving)

Calories: 25 Kcal; Total Carbohydrates: 6 g; Fiber: 2 g; Fat: 0 g; Protein: 0 g; Iron: 0 mg

*Pumpkin is a nice
change from squash.*

TIP

Dice extra pumpkin and freeze in a single layer on a baking sheet covered with plastic wrap. Once completely frozen, transfer to a resealable bag for use throughout the year.

Pumpkin

3 cups	cubed peeled pie pumpkin	750 mL
1 cup	water	250 mL

1. In a large saucepan, over medium-high heat, bring pumpkin and water to a boil. Cover, reduce heat and simmer until pumpkin is very tender, about 25 minutes. Let cool.

2. Transfer pumpkin and cooking liquid to blender and purée on high speed.

Nutritional Information (Per ¼-cup/50 mL Serving)

Calories: 8 Kcal; Total Carbohydrates: 2 g; Fiber: 0 g; Fat: 0 g; Protein: 0 g; Iron: 0 mg

Spinach

4 cups	lightly packed fresh spinach leaves (about 3 oz/90 g)	1 L
½ cup	water	125 mL

1. Wash spinach leaves thoroughly in a basin of cold water, changing water often. Remove tough stems and ribs and roughly chop leaves.

2. Arrange spinach in a large nonstick skillet. Pour in water, cover and cook over medium-high heat, stirring occasionally, until wilted and bright green, about 5 minutes. Let cool.

3. Transfer spinach to blender and purée on high speed.

Nutritional Information (Per ¼-cup/50 mL Serving)

Calories: 3 Kcal; Total Carbohydrates: 1 g; Fiber: 0 g; Fat: 0 g; Protein: 0 g; Iron: 0 mg

Squash

3 cups	cubed peeled butternut or acorn squash	750 mL
1 cup	water	250 mL

1. In a medium saucepan, over medium-high heat, bring squash and water to a boil. Cover, reduce heat and simmer until squash is very tender, about 20 minutes. Let cool.

2. Transfer squash to blender and purée on high speed.

Nutritional Information (Per ¼-cup/50 mL Serving)

Calories: 12 Kcal; Total Carbohydrates: 3 g; Fiber: 0 g; Fat: 0 g; Protein: 0 g; Iron: 0 mg

Sweet Peas

3 cups	fresh or frozen sweet peas	750 mL
2 cups	water	500 mL

MAKES ABOUT 2 CUPS (500 ML)

If shelling peas isn't quite the labor of love you were looking for, frozen peas offer the same nutritional value without the work

TIP

If your baby is texture-sensitive, push the purée through a fine sieve with a wooden spoon to get a very smooth consistency.

1. In a large saucepan, over medium-high heat, bring peas and water to a boil. Cover, reduce heat and simmer for 5 minutes, until peas are tender. Let cool.
2. Transfer peas to blender and purée on high speed.

> **Nutritional Information (Per ¼-cup/50 mL Serving)**
> Calories: 42 Kcal; Total Carbohydrates: 7 g; Fiber: 3 g; Fat: 0 g; Protein: 3 g; Iron: 1 mg

Sweet Potato

MAKES ABOUT 2 CUPS (500 ML)

Sweet potatoes, carrots, mangoes and other orange fruits and vegetables are high in beta carotene, which the body converts to vitamin A. Vitamin A is important for vision, bone growth, reproduction and cell division.

3 cups	cubed peeled sweet potatoes (about 2)	750 mL
1 cup	water	250 mL

1. In a medium saucepan, over medium-high heat, bring potatoes and water to a boil. Cover, reduce heat and simmer until potatoes are very tender, about 20 minutes. Let cool.
2. Transfer potatoes to blender and purée on high speed.

> **Nutritional Information (Per ¼-cup/50 mL Serving)**
> Calories: 26 Kcal; Total Carbohydrates: 6 g; Fiber: 1 g; Fat: 0 g; Protein: 0 g; Iron: 0 mg

**MAKES ABOUT
2 CUPS (500 ML)**

Turnips

| 2 cups | chopped peeled white turnips (about 4) | 500 mL |
| 1 cup | water | 250 mL |

1. In a medium saucepan, over medium-high heat, bring turnips and water to a boil. Cover, reduce heat and simmer until turnips are very tender, about 15 minutes. Let cool.

2. Transfer turnips to blender and purée on high speed.

> **Nutritional Information (Per ¼-cup/50 mL Serving)**
>
> Calories: 9 Kcal; Total Carbohydrates: 2 g; Fiber: 1 g; Fat: 0 g; Protein: 0 g; Iron: 0 mg

**MAKES ABOUT
2 CUPS (500 ML)**

Zucchini/Yellow Squash

| 3 cups | sliced zucchini or yellow squash (about 2) | 750 mL |

1. Place zucchini in a steaming basket fitted over a saucepan of boiling water, cover and steam for 15 minutes, or until very tender. Let cool.

2. Transfer zucchini to blender and purée on high speed.

> **Nutritional Information (Per ¼-cup/50 mL Serving)**
>
> Calories: 5 Kcal; Total Carbohydrates: 1 g; Fiber: 0 g; Fat: 0 g; Protein: 0 g; Iron: 0 mg

Apples, Plums and Cranberries

1 ½ cups	diced peeled apples (about 2)	375 mL
½ cup	sliced plum (about 1)	125 mL
½ cup	frozen apple juice concentrate	125 mL
¼ cup	fresh or frozen cranberries	50 mL

1. In a medium saucepan, over medium heat, bring apples, plum, apple juice concentrate and cranberries to a simmer. Cover, reduce heat and simmer until apples are very tender, about 20 minutes. Let cool.

2. Transfer to blender and purée on high speed.

> **Nutritional Information (Per ¼-cup/50 mL Serving)**
> Calories: 49 Kcal; Total Carbohydrates: 12 g; Fiber: 1 g;
> Fat: 0 g; Protein: 0 g; Iron: 0 mg

Cranberry Apple Mush

4 cups	sliced peeled apples (about 3 large)	1 L
½ cup	fresh or frozen cranberries	125 mL
½ cup	sweetened apple juice	125 mL
1 tsp	ground cinnamon	5 mL

1. In a medium saucepan, over medium-high heat, bring apples, cranberries, apple juice and cinnamon to a boil. Cover, reduce heat and simmer until apples are very tender, about 25 minutes. Let cool.

2. Transfer to blender and purée on high speed.

> **Nutritional Information (Per ¼-cup/50 mL Serving)**
> Calories: 44 Kcal; Total Carbohydrates: 11 g; Fiber: 2 g;
> Fat: 0 g; Protein: 0 g; Iron: 0 mg

Nectarines and Raspberries with Orange

MAKES ABOUT 2 CUPS (500 ML)

TIP

Substitute frozen raspberries when fresh are not in season.

FOR OLDER KIDS

Freeze mixture in ice-pop molds for a chilly treat.

2 cups	sliced nectarines (about 3)	500 mL
¼ cup	raspberries	50 mL
¼ cup	frozen orange juice concentrate	50 mL

1. In blender, on high speed, purée nectarines, raspberries and orange juice.

Nutritional Information (Per ¼-cup/50 mL Serving)

Calories: 33 Kcal; Total Carbohydrates: 8 g; Fiber: 1 g; Fat: 0 g; Protein: 1 g; Iron: 0 mg

Orange, Orange, Orange

MAKES ABOUT 2 CUPS (500 ML)

A deep orange color is generally an indication that the fruit or vegetable contains beta carotene and vitamin C— this is a triple dose, packed with flavor!

TIP

Substitute additional water for the orange juice for young stomachs that are irritated by citrus.

1 cup	diced peeled carrots (about 2)	250 mL
1 cup	diced peeled sweet potato (about ½)	250 mL
½ cup	diced peeled pear (about ½)	125 mL
½ cup	orange juice (see tip, at left)	125 mL
½ cup	water	125 mL

1. In a medium saucepan, over medium-high heat, bring carrots, sweet potato, pear, orange juice and water to a boil. Cover, reduce heat and simmer until vegetables are very tender, about 20 minutes. Let cool.

2. Transfer to blender with cooking liquid and purée on high speed, adding more water if necessary.

Nutritional Information (Per ¼-cup/50 mL Serving)

Calories: 71 Kcal; Total Carbohydrates: 12 g; Fiber: 1 g; Fat: 2 g; Protein: 1 g; Iron: 0 mg

**MAKES ABOUT
2 CUPS (500 ML)**

Summer fruits are combined in this quick and easy dessert.

TIP

Buy pitted cherries during the summer and keep them portioned in your freezer for easy use throughout the year.

FOR OLDER KIDS

Freeze mixture in ice-pop molds for a chilly treat.

Cherried Peaches

2 cups	sliced peeled peaches (about 3)	500 mL
1 cup	pitted red sour cherries (about 8 oz/250 g)	250 mL
½ cup	peach nectar	125 mL

1. In blender, on high speed, purée peaches, cherries and peach nectar.

Nutritional Information (Per ¼-cup/50 mL Serving)

Calories: 36 Kcal; Total Carbohydrates: 9 g; Fiber: 1 g; Fat: 0 g; Protein: 1 g; Iron: 0 mg

---

**MAKES ABOUT
3 CUPS (750 ML)**

FOR OLDER KIDS

For a special treat, stir this purée into their favorite porridge with a sprinkle of ground cinnamon.

Peach and Pear Bananarama

1½ cups	diced peeled peaches (about 2)	375 mL
1 cup	diced peeled pear (about 1)	250 mL
1	banana, sliced	1

1. In blender, on high speed, purée peaches, pear and banana.

Nutritional Information (Per ¼-cup/50 mL Serving)

Calories: 29 Kcal; Total Carbohydrates: 7 g; Fiber: 1 g; Fat: 0 g; Protein: 0 g; Iron: 0 mg

Figgy Pears

*Figs are a good source
of potassium and fiber;
paired with the mild,
sweet taste of pears
(which are also a good
source of soluble fiber)
this purée is a great
spread for adults too!*

1½ cups	diced peeled pears (about 2)	375 mL
¾ cup	unsweetened orange juice	175 mL
½ cup	diced figs, stems removed (about 4 oz/125 g)	125 mL
¼ tsp	ground allspice	1 mL

1. In a medium saucepan, over medium-low heat, combine pears, orange juice, figs and allspice. Bring to a simmer, cover and cook until pears and figs are very tender, about 20 minutes. Let cool.

2. Transfer to blender and purée on high speed.

Nutritional Information (Per ¼-cup/50 mL Serving)

Calories: 44 Kcal; Total Carbohydrates: 11 g; Fiber: 1 g; Fat: 0 g; Protein: 0 g; Iron: 0 mg

Purple Pears

*This smooth, deep
purple purée is sure
to be a hit, but be
aware that beets often
discolor urine and
stools. This is not
cause for concern.*

TIP

Avoid buying elongated
beets — they are
more fibrous and
do not provide a
smooth-textured purée.

1 cup	diced peeled beets (about 2)	250 mL
1 cup	diced peeled pear (about 1)	250 mL
½ cup	unsweetened apple juice	125 mL

1. In a medium saucepan, over low heat, combine beets, pear and apple juice. Bring to a simmer, cover and cook until beets and pears are very tender, about 30 minutes. Let cool.

2. Transfer to blender with cooking liquid and purée on high speed.

Nutritional Information (Per ¼-cup/50 mL Serving)

Calories: 27 Kcal; Total Carbohydrates: 7 g; Fiber: 1 g; Fat: 0 g; Protein: 0 g; Iron: 0 mg

**MAKES ABOUT
2 CUPS (500 ML)**

Plums with Orange and Lemon

3 cups	sliced plums (about 6)	750 mL
¼ cup	frozen orange juice concentrate	50 mL
	Grated zest and juice of 1 lemon	

1. In a medium saucepan, over medium-low heat, combine plums, orange juice concentrate, and lemon zest and juice. Bring to a simmer, cover and cook, stirring occasionally, until plums are very soft and can be broken up easily with fork, about 30 minutes. Let cool.

2. Transfer to blender and purée on high speed.

Nutritional Information (Per ¼-cup/50 mL Serving)

Calories: 50 Kcal; Total Carbohydrates: 12 g; Fiber: 1 g; Fat: 0 g; Protein: 1 g; Iron: 0 mg

**MAKES ABOUT
2 CUPS (500 ML)**

Blended melon flavors combine in a refreshing treat for your baby.

FOR OLDER KIDS

Freeze unused chopped peeled melon in an airtight container in the freezer. In blender, combine 1 cup (250 mL) frozen melon pieces and purée on high speed until smooth for an icy treat.

Melon Madness

1 cup	diced cantaloupe	250 mL
1 cup	diced honeydew melon	250 mL
1 cup	diced seedless watermelon	250 mL

1. In blender, on high speed, purée cantaloupe, honeydew and watermelon.

Nutritional Information (Per ¼-cup/50 mL Serving)

Calories: 21 Kcal; Total Carbohydrates: 5 g; Fiber: 0 g; Fat: 0 g; Protein: 0 g; Iron: 0 mg

Watermelon Refresher

*Watermelon blends
well with other fruits
to make a naturally
sweet thirst quencher.*

TIP

Use an equal amount
of frozen strawberries
when fresh are not
in season.

FOR OLDER KIDS

Freeze purée in
ice-pop molds for
a frosty treat.

2 cups	diced seedless watermelon	500 mL
½ cup	diced peeled kiwi (about 1)	125 mL
½ cup	sliced strawberries	125 mL
1 tbsp	lime juice	15 mL

1. In blender, on high speed, purée watermelon, kiwi, strawberries and lime juice.

Nutritional Information (Per ¼-cup/50 mL Serving)

Calories: 22 Kcal; Total Carbohydrates: 5 g; Fiber: 1 g; Fat: 0 g; Protein: 0 g; Iron: 0 mg

Rhubarb, Apples and Berries

TIP

Use an equal
amount of frozen
berries and rhubarb
when fresh are not
in season.

2 cups	sliced peeled apples (about 2)	500 mL
1 cup	chopped rhubarb (about 2 stalks)	250 mL
¼ cup	raspberries and/or blueberries	50 mL
¼ cup	frozen apple juice concentrate	50 mL

1. In a medium saucepan, over medium-low heat, combine apples, rhubarb, berries and apple juice concentrate. Bring to a simmer, cover and cook, stirring occasionally, until fruit is very tender, about 30 minutes. Let cool.

2. Transfer to blender and purée on high speed.

Nutritional Information (Per ¼-cup/50 mL Serving)

Calories: 36 Kcal; Total Carbohydrates: 9 g; Fiber: 1 g; Fat: 0 g; Protein: 0 g; Iron: 0 mg

Strawberry Decadence

**MAKES ABOUT
2 CUPS (500 ML)**

*Creamy apricots make
this strawberry purée
an absolute delight!*

TIP

Apricots are an
excellent source of
Vitamin A. When
fresh are not in
season, used dried
that have been
rehydrated in boiling
water for 30 minutes,
or until swollen and
softened. Use liquid
with apricots.

1 cup	fresh or frozen strawberries	250 mL
1 cup	sliced apricots (2 to 3)	250 mL
	Zest and juice of 1 lemon	

1. In blender, on high speed, purée strawberries, apricots, and lemon zest and juice.

2. *Make ahead:* Store in an airtight container in the refrigerator for up to 1 week.

> **Nutritional Information (Per ¼-cup/50 mL Serving)**
>
> Calories: 17 Kcal; Total Carbohydrates: 4 g; Fiber: 1 g; Fat: 0 g; Protein: 0 g; Iron: 0 mg

Tropical Fruit Breeze

**MAKES ABOUT
2 CUPS (500 ML)**

FOR OLDER KIDS

To make a great
smoothie, add ½ cup
(125 mL) milk to
1 cup (250 mL) of
the purée.

1 cup	chopped peeled kiwi (about 2)	250 mL
1	sliced banana (about 1 small)	125 mL
½ cup	chopped peeled mango (about ½)	125 mL
½ cup	orange juice	125 mL

1. In blender, on high speed, purée kiwi, banana, mango and orange juice.

2. *Make ahead:* Store in the refrigerator for up to 5 days.

> **Nutritional Information (Per ½-cup/125 mL Serving)**
>
> Calories: 107 Kcal; Total Carbohydrates: 27 g; Fiber: 3 g; Fat: 1 g; Protein: 1 g; Iron: 0 mg; Vitamin C: 54 mg

Fruit Explosion

TIP

Use equal amounts of frozen peaches and blueberries when fresh are not in season.

FOR OLDER KIDS

Stir ¼ cup (50 mL) of the fruit compote into oatmeal or yogurt and sprinkle with ground cinnamon.

1 cup	sliced peeled peaches (1 to 2)	250 mL
1	small banana	1
½ cup	blueberries	125 mL
½ cup	unsweetened applesauce	125 mL

1. In blender, on high speed, purée peaches, banana, blueberries and applesauce. Pass through a fine sieve with a wooden spoon to remove seeds.

Nutritional Information (Per ¼-cup/50 mL Serving)

Calories: 29 Kcal; Total Carbohydrates: 8 g; Fiber: 1 g; Fat: 0 g; Protein: 0 g; Iron: 0 mg

Avocado, Mango and Lime

TIPS

Avocados offer more protein than any other fruit and are high in essential fatty acids, ideal for baby's development.

Prevent discoloration of the avocado's flesh by sprinkling it with lemon or lime juice.

½ cup	diced peeled avocado (about ½)	125 mL
½ cup	diced peeled mango (about ½)	125 mL
2 tbsp	freshly squeezed lime juice	25 mL

1. In blender, on high speed, purée avocado, mango and lime juice.

2. *Make ahead:* Store in the refrigerator for up to 1 day.

Nutritional Information (Per ¼-cup/50 mL Serving)

Calories: 44 Kcal; Total Carbohydrates: 5 g; Fiber: 1 g; Fat: 3 g; Protein: 0 g; Iron: 0 mg

Carrots and Dates

MAKES ABOUT 2 CUPS (500 ML)

Dates lend sweetness and fiber to a favorite vegetable!

TIP

Use this as a spread on whole-grain toast and bran muffins for the whole family.

2 cups	sliced peeled carrots (about 4)	500 mL
1 cup	unsweetened apple juice or water	250 mL
½ cup	chopped pitted dates (about 3 oz/90 g)	125 mL

1. In a medium saucepan, over medium-high heat, bring carrots, apple juice and dates to a boil. Cover, reduce heat and simmer until carrots are very tender, about 15 minutes. Let cool.

2. Transfer to blender and purée on high speed.

Nutritional Information (Per ¼-cup/50 mL Serving)

Calories: 52 Kcal; Total Carbohydrates: 13 g; Fiber: 1 g; Fat: 0 g; Protein: 0 g; Iron: 0 mg

Carrots with Apricots and Berries

MAKES ABOUT 2 CUPS (500 ML)

TIP

Use an equal amount of frozen raspberries when fresh are not in season.

1 cup	diced peeled carrots (about 2)	250 mL
1 cup	sliced pitted apricots (2 to 3)	250 mL
½ cup	raspberries	125 mL

1. Place carrots in a steaming basket fitted over a saucepan of boiling water; cover and steam until very tender, about 15 minutes. Let cool.

2. Transfer to blender, add carrots, apricots and raspberries; purée on high speed. Pass through a fine sieve with a wooden spoon to remove seeds.

Nutritional Information (Per ¼-cup/50 mL Serving)

Calories: 20 Kcal; Total Carbohydrates: 5 g; Fiber: 1 g; Fat: 0 g; Protein: 1 g; Iron: 0 mg

**MAKES ABOUT
2 CUPS (500 ML)**

Combining fruits and veggies is a great way to pack nutrients into simple purées.

Pears, Carrots and Squash

1 cup	diced peeled butternut squash	250 mL
1 cup	sliced peeled pear (about 1)	250 mL
½ cup	sliced peeled carrot (about 1)	125 mL
¼ cup	unsweetened apple juice or water	50 mL

1. In a medium saucepan, over medium heat, combine squash, pear, carrot and apple juice. Bring to a simmer, cover and cook until all are very tender, about 20 minutes. Let cool.

2. Transfer to blender and purée on high speed.

Nutritional Information (Per ¼-cup/50 mL Serving)

Calories: 24 Kcal; Total Carbohydrates: 6 g; Fiber: 1 g; Fat: 0 g; Protein: 0 g; Iron: 0 mg

---

**MAKES ABOUT
2 CUPS (500 ML)**

Pumpkin and Apples

2 cups	cubed peeled apples (about 2)	500 mL
1 cup	diced peeled pie pumpkin	250 mL
½ cup	unsweetened apple juice	125 mL
1 tsp	vanilla	5 mL
½ tsp	ground cinnamon	2 mL

1. In a medium saucepan, over medium-low heat, combine apples, pumpkin, apple juice, vanilla and cinnamon. Cover and simmer until apples and pumpkin are very tender, about 30 minutes. Let cool.

2. Transfer to blender and purée on high speed.

Nutritional Information (Per ¼-cup/50 mL Serving)

Calories: 22 Kcal; Total Carbohydrates: 5 g; Fiber: 1 g; Fat: 0 g; Protein: 1 g; Iron: 0 mg

Pumpkin has more flavor than other varieties of winter squash; it's a nice alternative when in season.

TIPS

Do not substitute canned pie filling, which has additives in it, for the pumpkin.

Cut peeled and seeded pumpkin into chunks and freeze in a resealable bag for up to 6 months.

Orange Pumpkin Purée

- Preheat oven to 350°F (180°C)
- Rimmed baking sheet, lined with foil

2 cups	cubed peeled pie pumpkin	500 mL
1 tbsp	vegetable oil	15 mL
1 tsp	ground cinnamon	5 mL
Pinch	ground allspice	Pinch
½ cup	orange juice	125 mL

1. In a medium bowl, toss pumpkin with vegetable oil, cinnamon and allspice.

2. Arrange in a single layer on prepared baking sheet and bake in preheated oven until pumpkin is golden and tender, about 30 minutes. Let cool slightly.

3. Transfer to blender, add orange juice and purée on high speed.

Nutritional Information (Per ¼-cup/50 mL Serving)

Calories: 30 Kcal; Total Carbohydrates: 4 g; Fiber: 0 g; Fat: 2 g; Protein: 0 g; Iron: 0 mg

---

*Although it may
seem like an odd
combination, this
purée is nutritious
and delicious!*

TIP

Summer squash
varieties such as
zucchini should
either be steamed
or cooked in a very
small amount of water
— they become too
watery when boiled.

Zucchini and Nectarines

1 ½ cups	sliced nectarines (about 2)	375 mL
1 cup	sliced zucchini (about 1 small)	250 mL
¼ cup	water	50 mL

1. In a medium saucepan, over medium-low heat, combine nectarines, zucchini and water. Bring to a simmer, cover and cook until zucchini and nectarines are very tender, about 20 minutes. Let cool.

2. Transfer zucchini and nectarines to blender and purée on high speed.

Nutritional Information (Per ¼-cup/50 mL Serving)

Calories: 12 Kcal; Total Carbohydrates: 3 g; Fiber: 1 g; Fat: 0 g; Protein: 0 g; Iron: 0 mg

---

*Taste the fall
harvest in this rich
vegetable purée!*

Squashed Green Beans

1 cup	diced peeled butternut squash	250 mL
½ cup	unsweetened apple juice or water	125 mL
1 ½ cups	sliced trimmed green beans	375 mL

1. In a medium saucepan, over medium-high heat, combine squash and apple juice. Add enough water to completely cover squash. Cover and bring to a boil; reduce heat and simmer for 10 minutes. Add green beans, cover and cook until beans and squash are very tender, about 10 minutes. Let cool.

2. Transfer to blender with cooking liquid and purée on high speed.

Nutritional Information (Per ¼-cup/50 mL Serving)

Calories: 43 Kcal; Total Carbohydrates: 11 g; Fiber: 2 g; Fat: 0 g; Protein: 1 g; Iron 1 mg

**MAKES ABOUT
2 CUPS (500 ML)**

*Sweet and mild root
vegetables team up in
this tasty purée!*

Celery Root, Carrots and Parsnips

1 cup	cubed peeled carrots (about 2)	250 mL
½ cup	cubed peeled celery root	125 mL
½ cup	cubed peeled parsnip (about 1)	125 mL

1. In a medium saucepan, over medium-high heat, combine carrots, celery root and parsnip. Pour in enough water just to cover. Bring to a boil. Cover, reduce heat and simmer until all vegetable are very tender, about 15 minutes. Let cool.

2. Transfer to blender with cooking liquid and purée on high speed.

Nutritional Information (Per ¼-cup/50 mL Serving)

Calories: 14 Kcal; Total Carbohydrates: 3 g; Fiber: 1 g; Fat: 0 g; Protein: 0 g; Iron: 0 mg

**MAKES ABOUT
2 CUPS (500 ML)**

Yummy Broccoli

3 cups	broccoli florets	750 mL
½ cup	unsweetened apple juice or water	125 mL

1. Place broccoli in a steaming basket fitted over a saucepan of boiling water. Cover and steam until broccoli is very tender, about 15 to 20 minutes. Let cool.

2. Transfer broccoli to blender, add apple juice and purée on high speed.

Nutritional Information (Per ¼-cup/50 mL Serving)

Calories: 22 Kcal; Total Carbohydrates: 5 g; Fiber: 1 g; Fat: 0 g; Protein: 1 g; Iron: 0 mg; Vitamin C: 25 mg

MAKES ABOUT
2 CUPS (500 ML)

Molasses adds iron and a hint of sweetness to two favorites.

TIPS

There are many types of molasses available, but blackstrap has the least amount of sugar and the most nutrients.

Sweet potatoes are a good source of beta carotene.

Corny Sweet Potatoes

1 1/2 cups	diced peeled sweet potato (about 1)	375 mL
1 cup	corn kernels	250 mL
1/4 cup	orange juice	50 mL
1 tbsp	blackstrap molasses	15 mL

1. Place sweet potato in a steaming basket fitted over a saucepan of boiling water. Cover and steam until very tender, about 20 minutes. Add corn and steam for 2 minutes longer. Let cool.

2. Transfer sweet potato and corn to blender and add orange juice and molasses; purée on high speed.

Nutritional Information (Per 1/4-cup/50 mL Serving)

Calories: 53 Kcal; Total Carbohydrates: 12 g; Fiber: 1 g; Fat: 0 g; Protein: 1 g; Iron: 0 mg

MAKES ABOUT
2 CUPS (500 ML)

Pairing broccoli with the mild, sweet flavors of squash and carrots is a great way to introduce it.

TIP

Cut vegetables into equal-sized pieces for even cooking and cook until they break apart when pierced with a fork; this will ensure the smoothest consistency when the vegetables are puréed.

Squashed Vegetable Purée

1 cup	diced peeled butternut squash	250 mL
1/2 cup	sliced peeled broccoli stems	125 mL
1/2 cup	diced peeled carrot (about 1)	125 mL
1/4 cup	orange juice	50 mL

1. Place squash, broccoli stems and carrots in a steaming basket fitted over a saucepan of boiling water. Cover and steam for 15 to 20 minutes, or until very tender. Let cool.

2. Transfer vegetables to blender, add orange juice, and purée on high speed.

Nutritional Information (Per 1/4-cup/50 mL Serving)

Calories: 16 Kcal; Total Carbohydrates: 4 g; Fiber: 1 g; Fat: 0 g; Protein: 0 g; Iron: 0 mg

**MAKES ABOUT
4 CUPS (1 L)**

Vegetable Medley

1 cup	sliced trimmed green beans	250 mL
1 cup	sliced peeled carrots (about 2)	250 mL
½ cup	corn kernels	125 mL
½ cup	broccoli florets	125 mL
½ cup	cauliflower florets	125 mL
½ cup	canned diced tomatoes, with juice	125 mL

1. Place green beans, carrots, corn, broccoli and cauliflower in a steaming basket fitted over a saucepan of boiling water. Cover and steam until vegetables are very tender, about 20 minutes. Let cool.

2. Transfer vegetables to blender, add tomatoes with juice and purée on high speed, adding water if necessary, until smooth.

Nutritional Information (Per ¼-cup/50 mL Serving)

Calories: 13 Kcal; Total Carbohydrates: 3 g; Fiber: 1 g; Fat: 0 g; Protein: 1 g; Iron: 0 mg

**MAKES ABOUT
1 CUP (125 ML)**

FOR OLDER KIDS

Serve as a dip with baked whole wheat tortilla or pita wedges.

Guacamole for Beginners

1 cup	sliced peeled avocado (about 1)	250 mL
½ cup	chopped peeled and seeded tomato	125 mL
2 tbsp	freshly squeezed lime juice	25 mL

1. In blender, combine avocado, tomato and lime juice and purée on high speed until smooth.

2. *Make ahead:* Store in an airtight container in the refrigerator for up to 3 days. Do not freeze.

Nutritional Information (Per ¼-cup/50 mL Serving)

Calories: 65 Kcal; Total Carbohydrates: 4 g; Fiber: 1 g; Fat: 6 g; Protein: 1 g; Iron: 0 mg

**MAKES ABOUT
2 CUPS (500 ML)**

Zucchini and White Beans

1	zucchini, sliced	1
1 cup	rinsed and drained canned white beans	250 mL
1 cup	low-sodium vegetable stock	250 mL

1. In a medium saucepan, over medium-low heat, combine zucchini, beans and stock; bring to a simmer. Cover and simmer until zucchini is very tender, about 15 minutes. Let cool.

2. Transfer to blender and purée on high speed.

Nutritional Information (Per $\frac{1}{2}$-cup/125 mL Serving)

Calories: 93 Kcal; Total Carbohydrates: 16 g; Fiber: 4 g; Fat: 0 g; Protein: 8 g; Iron: 3 mg

---

**MAKES 1 CUP
(250 ML)**

FOR OLDER KIDS

Serve as a dip for vegetables and strips of baked whole wheat pitas.

Hummus for Beginners

1 cup	rinsed and drained canned chickpeas	250 mL
$\frac{1}{2}$ cup	water	125 mL

1. In blender, on high speed, purée chickpeas.

2. *Make ahead:* Store in the refrigerator for up to 3 days. Do not freeze.

Nutritional Information (Per $\frac{1}{4}$-cup/50 mL Serving)

Calories: 71 Kcal; Total Carbohydrates: 14 g; Fiber: 3 g; Fat: 1 g; Protein: 3 g; Iron: 1 mg

**MAKES ABOUT
2 CUPS (500 ML)**

This intensely colored purée is packed full of delicious nutrients.

TIP

Lentils do not have to be soaked, but rinse well in a sieve and pick through to remove any small stones.

FOR OLDER KIDS

Serve as a dip with warm naan bread or whole wheat pita wedges.

Dhal for Beginners

1 ½ cups	low-sodium vegetable stock	375 mL
¼ cup	dried red lentils, rinsed	50 mL
½ tsp	ground coriander	2 mL
¼ tsp	ground turmeric	1 mL
1	small potato, peeled and diced	1
1	carrot, peeled and diced	1
½ cup	cauliflower florets	125 mL

1. In a medium saucepan, combine stock, lentils, coriander and turmeric; bring to a boil. Cover, reduce heat and simmer for 15 minutes, until lentils are slightly tender.

2. Stir in potato, carrot and cauliflower; cover and simmer until vegetables and lentils are very tender, about 15 minutes. Let cool.

3. Transfer to blender and purée on high speed.

> **Nutritional Information (Per ¼-cup/50 mL Serving)**
>
> Calories: 84 Kcal; Total Carbohydrates: 13 g; Fiber: 6 g; Fat: 0 g; Protein: 8 g; Iron: 2 mg

**MAKES ABOUT
2 CUPS (500 ML)**

Lean white fish has a very mild flavor and can be quickly prepared.

FOR OLDER KIDS

Spoon ½ cup (125 mL) purée onto a split baked potato and sprinkle with shredded cheese. Bake in preheated 350°F (180°C) oven until potato is warmed through and cheese is melted, about 15 minutes.

Fish and Mushy Peas

1 cup	frozen sweet peas	250 mL
6 oz	skinless cod,* haddock or halibut fillet	175 g
½ cup	low-sodium vegetable stock	125 mL
1 tsp	freshly squeezed lemon juice	5 mL

* Nutritional information is for cod

1. Arrange peas in a medium saucepan. Place fish on top and pour stock over fish. Cover and cook over medium heat until fish flakes easily when tested with a fork, about 10 minutes. Let cool.

2. Transfer to blender, add lemon juice and blend on high speed to desired consistency.

Nutritional Information (Per ½-cup/125 mL Serving)

Calories: 69 Kcal; Total Carbohydrates: 5 g; Fiber: 2 g; Fat: 0 g; Protein: 11 g; Iron: 1 mg

**MAKES ABOUT
2 CUPS (500 ML)**

*Celery brings great
flavor to this
delicate dish.*

Cod with Celery and Peppers

6 oz	skinless cod fillet	175 g
1	stalk celery, diced	1
1 cup	diced red bell pepper	250 mL
1 cup	water	250 mL
1/4 cup	long-grain white rice	50 mL

1. In a medium saucepan, combine cod, celery, red pepper, water and rice; bring to a boil over medium-high heat. Cover, reduce heat and simmer until fish flakes easily when tested with a fork and rice is tender, about 15 minutes. Let cool.

2. Transfer to blender and blend on high speed to desired consistency.

Nutritional Information (Per 1/2-cup/125 mL Serving)

Calories: 90 Kcal; Total Carbohydrates: 12 g; Fiber: 1 g; Fat: 0 g; Protein: 9 g; Iron: 1 mg; Vitamin C: 72 mg

**MAKES ABOUT
2 CUPS (500 ML)**

*The mild flavor of
this purée is especially
pleasing to young
palates.*

TIP

Cooking the leek and
corn first gives them
a mild, sweet flavor. If
you're in a hurry, omit
the oil and cook the
leek, corn, fish and
water in a covered pot
over medium-high
heat until leek is
tender and fish flakes
easily when tested
with a fork, about
8 minutes. Purée
on high speed to
desired consistency.

Haddock, Corn and Leeks

2 tsp	olive oil	10 mL
1/2 cup	chopped leek, white and light green parts only	125 mL
1 cup	frozen sweet corn	250 mL
6 oz	skinless haddock fillet	175 g
1/4 cup	water	50 mL

1. In a nonstick skillet, heat oil over medium-high heat. Add leek and cook, stirring, until tender but not browned, about 3 minutes. Add corn and cook for 2 minutes more. Arrange haddock on top of leek-corn mixture and pour in water; cover and cook until fish flakes easily when tested with a fork, about 8 minutes. Let cool.

2. Transfer to blender and blend on high speed to desired consistency.

Nutritional Information (Per 1/2-cup/125 mL Serving)

Calories: 100 Kcal; Total Carbohydrates: 10 g; Fiber: 1 g; Fat: 3 g; Protein: 9 g; Iron: 1 mg

---

**MAKES ABOUT
2 CUPS (500 ML)**

*Oily fish, such as
salmon, are an
excellent source of
iron. Iron is absorbed
more easily when
combined with vitamin
C, which in this recipe
is provided by the
broccoli.*

Cheesy Salmon and Broccoli Dinner

1 cup	broccoli florets	250 mL
1	small potato, peeled and diced	1
8 oz	skinless salmon fillets	250 g
½ cup	homogenized (whole) milk	125 mL
¼ cup	shredded Cheddar cheese	50 mL

1. Arrange potatoes and broccoli in a medium saucepan. Lay salmon fillets on top and pour milk over salmon; bring to a boil over medium-high heat. Cover, reduce heat and simmer for 15 to 20 minutes, or until vegetables are tender and fish flakes easily when tested with a fork. Let cool.

2. Transfer to blender, add cheese and blend on high speed to desired consistency.

Nutritional Information (Per ½-cup/125 mL Serving)

Calories: 133 Kcal; Total Carbohydrates: 6 g; Fiber: 1 g;
Fat: 5 g; Protein: 15 g; Iron: 1 mg; Vitamin C: 21 mg

**MAKES ABOUT
2 CUPS (500 ML)**

Spinach, Salmon and Rice

2 tsp	olive oil	10 mL
¼ cup	chopped onion	50 mL
½ cup	long-grain white rice	125 mL
1 cup	water (approx.)	250 mL
1 cup	chopped fresh spinach	250 mL
4 oz	skinless salmon fillet	125 g
1 tsp	freshly squeezed lemon juice	5 mL

1. In a medium saucepan, heat oil over medium-high heat. Add onion and cook, stirring, until tender but not browned, about 3 minutes.

2. Add rice and stir until coated with oil. Stir in water and bring to a boil. Cover, reduce heat, and simmer until most of the water has been absorbed and rice is slightly tender, about 15 minutes.

3. Arrange spinach and salmon on top of rice; cover and continue to cook until spinach is wilted and salmon flakes easily when tested with a fork, about 10 minutes. Let sit, covered, for 10 minutes.

4. Transfer to blender, add lemon juice and blend on high speed to desired consistency, adding more water if necessary.

Variation

For the ultimate in nutritional density, substitute an equal amount of blanched Swiss chard for the spinach.

Nutritional Information (Per ½-cup/125 mL Serving)

Calories: 143 Kcal; Total Carbohydrates: 20 g; Fiber: 1 g; Fat: 3 g; Protein: 8 g; Iron: 1 mg

**MAKES ABOUT
2 CUPS (500 ML)**

*Brightly colored
vegetables abound in
this summertime feast!*

TIPS

Asparagus is an
excellent source of
vitamin E. It contains
a sulfurous substance
that can be smelled
in urine but has no
harmful effect.

Refrigerate unused
asparagus upright in
½ inch (1 cm) water
for up to 3 days to
maintain freshness.
Or blanch spears and
store in a resealable
bag in the freezer for
up to 9 months.

Summer Salmon Supper

● *Preheat oven to 350°F (180°C)*
● *Rimmed baking sheet, lined with foil*

4 oz	skinless salmon fillet	125 g
4	asparagus spears, chopped	4
1	yellow summer squash (zucchini), sliced	1
¼ tsp	dried dillweed	1 mL
½ tsp	freshly squeezed lemon juice	2 mL

1. Arrange salmon in the center of prepared baking sheet. Arrange asparagus and squash on top and sprinkle with dill and lemon juice. Cover tightly with foil and bake in the center of preheated oven for 10 to 12 minutes, or until salmon flakes easily when tested with a fork and vegetables are tender. Let cool.

2. Transfer to blender with pan juices and blend on high speed to desired consistency, adding water if necessary.

Nutritional Information (Per ½-cup/125 mL Serving)

Calories: 47 Kcal; Total Carbohydrates: 3 g; Fiber: 1 g; Fat: 1 g; Protein: 7 g; Iron: 1 mg

---

**MAKES ABOUT
2 CUPS (500 ML)**

Tilapia, Celery and Tomatoes

1 tbsp	olive oil	15 mL
1/2 cup	thinly sliced celery	125 mL
1/2 cup	sliced green onions	125 mL
1/2 cup	diced tomato	125 mL
1/2 tsp	dried dillweed	2 mL
4 oz	skinless tilapia fillet	175 g
1/2 cup	water	125 mL

1. In a medium saucepan, heat oil over medium-high heat. Add celery, green onions and tomato; cook, stirring occasionally, until celery is tender, about 5 minutes. Add tilapia and water; cover and cook until fish flakes easily when tested with a fork, about 5 minutes. Let cool.

2. Transfer to blender and purée on high speed.

Nutritional Information (Per 1/2-cup/125 mL Serving)

Calories: 64 Kcal; Total Carbohydrates: 3 g; Fiber: 1 g; Fat: 4 g; Protein: 6 g; Iron: 0 mg

---

**MAKES ABOUT
2 CUPS (500 ML)**

*The mild flavor of
zucchini blends well
with tender pink trout.*

TIP

The pink flesh of the
trout gives this savory
purée a beautiful
color, but other fish
can be substituted
and cooked in the
same manner.

Trout, Zucchini and Potatoes

1	medium Yukon gold potato, peeled and diced	1
1	zucchini, diced	1
6 oz	trout fillet	175 g
	Water	

1. Arrange potato and zucchini in a medium saucepan. Lay trout on top, skin side down, and add enough water to almost cover potato and zucchini; cover and bring to a boil over medium-high heat. Reduce heat and simmer until potatoes are tender and trout flakes easily when tested with a fork, about 15 minutes. Let cool.

2. Remove skin from trout. Transfer to blender with potato-zucchini mixture and cooking liquid; purée on high speed, adding more water if necessary.

Nutritional Information (Per $\frac{1}{2}$-cup/125 mL Serving)

Calories: 96 Kcal; Total Carbohydrates: 7 g; Fiber: 1 g; Fat: 3 g; Protein: 10 g; Iron: 1 mg

MAKES ABOUT 1½ CUPS (375 ML)

TIPS

Roasted or poached chicken can be blended in the same manner.

For better flavor, substitute an equal amount of low-sodium chicken stock for the water.

Chicken

| 8 oz | boneless skinless chicken breast, cut in strips | 250 g |
| 1 cup | water | 250 mL |

1. Arrange chicken in a steamer basket fitted over a saucepan of boiling water. Cover and steam until chicken is no longer pink inside, about 20 minutes. Let cool.
2. Transfer to blender, add water and blend on high speed to desired consistency.

> **Nutritional Information (Per ¼-cup/50 mL Serving)**
>
> Calories: 50 Kcal; Total Carbohydrates: 0 g; Fiber: 0 g; Fat: 1 g; Protein: 10 g; Iron: 1 mg

MAKES ABOUT 2 CUPS (500 ML)

Kids love the mild flavors of chicken and celery.

TIP

For a smooth purée, remove the tough fibers from the celery ribs before chopping.

FOR OLDER KIDS

Stir purée into cooked brown rice for a quick meal.

Chicken with Celery

6 oz	boneless skinless chicken breast, diced	175 g
1 cup	chopped celery	250 mL
1 cup	low-sodium chicken stock	250 mL

1. In a medium saucepan, combine chicken, celery and stock; bring to a simmer over medium heat. Cover and simmer until celery is very tender and chicken is no longer pink inside, about 15 minutes. Let cool.
2. Transfer to blender and purée on high speed.

> **Nutritional Information (Per ½-cup/125 mL Serving)**
>
> Calories: 42 Kcal; Total Carbohydrates: 2 g; Fiber: 1 g; Fat: 0 g; Protein: 8 g; Iron: 1 mg

**MAKES ABOUT
2 CUPS (500 ML)**

*Roasted red pepper
adds smoky sweetness
to chicken and corn.*

Chicken with
Red Peppers and Corn

1 tbsp	olive oil	15 mL
6 oz	boneless skinless chicken breast, chopped	175 g
¼ cup	chopped onion	50 mL
½ cup	chopped roasted red bell pepper	125 mL
½ cup	frozen sweet corn	125 mL
1 tbsp	chopped fresh parsley	15 mL
½ cup	low-sodium chicken stock	125 mL

1. In a skillet, heat oil over medium-high heat. Add chicken, turning to brown evenly; transfer to a plate.

2. Add onion to skillet and cook, stirring, until tender, about 5 minutes. Stir in pepper, corn and parsley; cook for 2 minutes. Add stock and bring to a boil. Add browned chicken; cover, reduce heat and simmer until chicken is no longer pink inside and sauce thickens slightly. Let cool.

3. Transfer to blender and blend on high speed to desired consistency.

Nutritional Information (Per ½-cup/125 mL Serving)

Calories: 110 Kcal; Total Carbohydrates: 6 g; Fiber: 1 g; Fat: 5 g; Protein: 12 g; Iron: 1 mg; Vitamin C: 15 mg

---

Avocado with Chicken

**MAKES ABOUT
2 CUPS (500 ML)**

TIP

Cooking time depends
on the thickness of
the chicken breast.

FOR OLDER KIDS

Serve as a dip with
baked whole wheat
tortilla wedges.

8 oz	boneless skinless chicken breast, cut in strips	250 g
1	avocado, peeled, pitted and sliced	1
1 tbsp	freshly squeezed lime juice	15 mL
¾ cup	low-sodium chicken stock	175 mL

1. Arrange chicken in a steamer basket fitted over a saucepan of boiling water. Cover and steam for 10 to 15 minutes, until chicken is no longer pink inside. Transfer to a cutting board and cut into 1-inch (2.5 cm) pieces. Let cool.

2. Transfer to blender and add avocado, lime juice and stock; blend on high speed to desired consistency.

3. *Make ahead*: Store in the refrigerator for up to 3 days. Do not freeze.

Nutritional Information (Per ½-cup/125 mL Serving)

Calories: 119 Kcal; Total Carbohydrates: 3 g; Fiber: 1 g; Fat: 7 g; Protein: 12 g; Iron: 1 mg

---

**MAKES ABOUT
2 CUPS (500 ML)**

Chicken with Pumpkin

1 tbsp	olive oil	15 mL
6 oz	boneless skinless chicken breast, diced	175 g
1 cup	cubed peeled pie pumpkin	250 mL
1/2 cup	low-sodium chicken stock	125 mL
1/2 tsp	ground cinnamon	2 mL
1/4 tsp	ground allspice	1 mL
1/4 tsp	ground ginger	1 mL

1. In a medium saucepan, heat oil over medium heat. Add chicken, turning to brown evenly. Stir in pumpkin, stock, cinnamon, allspice and ginger; bring to a boil. Cover, reduce heat and simmer until chicken is no longer pink inside and pumpkin is very tender, about 20 minutes. Let cool.

2. Transfer to blender and purée on high speed.

Nutritional Information (Per 1/2-cup/125 mL Serving)

Calories: 70 Kcal; Total Carbohydrates: 3 g; Fiber: 0 g;
Fat: 4 g; Protein: 7 g; Iron: 1 mg

Chicken with Brown Rice and Peas

MAKES ABOUT 2 CUPS (500 ML)

A small amount of curry powder provides taste without heat, and will give little ones a palate for flavor!

TIP

Use whole-grain products such as brown rice and whole wheat bread to increase daily fiber intake.

1 tbsp	olive oil	15 mL
6 oz	boneless skinless chicken thighs, chopped	175 g
½ cup	chopped onion	125 mL
½ tsp	curry powder	2 mL
1½ cups	low-sodium chicken stock	375 mL
½ cup	long-grain brown rice, rinsed	125 mL
1 cup	frozen sweet peas	250 mL

1. In a medium saucepan, heat oil over medium-high heat. Add chicken, turning to brown evenly; transfer to a plate.

2. Add onion and curry powder to saucepan; cook, stirring, until onion is tender but not browned, about 3 minutes. Stir in stock and rice; bring to a boil. Cover, reduce heat and simmer for 25 to 30 minutes, or until rice is almost tender. Add peas and browned chicken; simmer until chicken is no longer pink inside, about 10 minutes. Let cool.

3. Transfer to blender and blend on high speed to desired consistency.

Nutritional Information (Per ½-cup/125 mL Serving)

Calories: 193 Kcal; Total Carbohydrates: 26 g; Fiber: 3 g; Fat: 5 g; Protein: 11 g; Iron: 2 mg

**MAKES ABOUT
2 CUPS (500 ML)**

Chicken Divine

1 tbsp	vegetable oil	15 mL
6 oz	boneless skinless chicken breast or thighs, chopped	175 g
½ cup	chopped onion	125 mL
½ cup	sliced white mushrooms	125 mL
1 cup	broccoli florets	250 mL
¼ cup	shredded Cheddar cheese	50 mL

1. In a nonstick skillet, heat oil over medium-high heat. Add chicken, turning to brown evenly; transfer to a plate.

2. Add onion to skillet and cook, stirring, until tender, about 5 minutes. Add mushrooms and cook, stirring, until golden, about 7 minutes. Add water, broccoli and browned chicken; bring just to a boil. Cover, reduce heat and simmer until broccoli is very tender and chicken is no longer pink inside, about 10 minutes. Let cool.

3. Transfer to blender, sprinkle with cheese and blend on high speed to desired consistency.

Nutritional Information (Per ½-cup/125 mL Serving)

Calories: 132 Kcal; Total Carbohydrates: 3 g; Fiber: 1 g; Fat: 9 g; Protein: 10 g; Iron: 1 mg; Vitamin C: 18 mg

**MAKES ABOUT
2 CUPS (500 ML)**

*Ripe mango provides
vitamins A and C
and gives a mild,
sweet flavor to this
protein-rich dish.
Mango skin can
irritate a baby's
mouth, so always
peel before using.*

TIP

Mangoes with
shriveled skin tend
to have fibrous flesh
that is very acidic and
unpleasant-tasting.
Ripe mangoes have a
sweet, fragrant aroma
and yield slightly
to the touch.

Tropical Chicken

1 tbsp	vegetable oil	15 mL
¼ cup	diced onion	50 mL
6 oz	boneless skinless chicken breast, chopped	175 g
¼ cup	long-grain brown rice, rinsed	50 mL
½ cup	low-sodium chicken stock	125 mL
½ cup	diced peeled mango	125 mL

1. In a medium saucepan, heat oil over medium-high heat. Add onion and cook, stirring, until tender but not browned, about 5 minutes. Add chicken and cook, stirring, until lightly browned, about 7 minutes. Stir in rice and cook for 1 minute more. Stir in stock and mango; bring to a boil. Cover, reduce heat and simmer until rice is tender and chicken is no longer pink inside, about 40 minutes. Let cool.

2. Transfer to blender and blend on high speed to desired consistency.

Nutritional Information (Per ½-cup/125 mL Serving)

Calories: 127 Kcal; Total Carbohydrates: 13 g; Fiber: 1 g; Fat: 2 g; Protein: 13 g; Iron: 1 mg

---

*Classic comfort food
for your baby!*

FOR OLDER KIDS

Put $1/2$ cup (125 mL)
purée in a ramekin or
gratin dish. Use
refrigerated dinner-roll
dough (cut to fit) to
cover, using excess
to form your child's
initial and place on
top. Bake in preheated
350°F (180°C) oven
until pastry is golden
and filling is warm,
about 12 minutes.

Chicken Stew

1 tbsp	vegetable oil	15 mL
6 oz	boneless skinless chicken breast, chopped	175 g
$1/2$ cup	diced peeled carrot	125 mL
$1/4$ cup	diced onion	50 mL
$1/4$ cup	diced celery	50 mL
1	small potato, cubed	1
1 cup	low-sodium chicken stock	250 mL
1 tbsp	minced fresh parsley	15 mL

1. In a medium saucepan, heat oil over medium-high heat. Add chicken, turning to brown evenly; transfer to a plate.

2. Add carrot, onion and celery to saucepan; cook until tender but not browned, about 5 minutes. Stir in potato and stock; bring to a boil. Return browned chicken to pan. Cover, reduce heat and simmer until potatoes are very tender and chicken is no longer pink inside, about 20 minutes. Stir in parsley. Let cool.

3. Transfer to blender and blend on high speed to desired consistency.

Nutritional Information (Per $1/2$-cup/125 mL Serving)

Calories: 120 Kcal; Total Carbohydrates: 7 g; Fiber: 1 g; Fat: 4 g; Protein: 14 g; Iron: 1 mg

Turkey with Cranberries

**MAKES ABOUT
2 CUPS (500 ML)**

*Don't leave your
little one out over
the holidays!*

TIPS

Use 1 cup (250 mL)
chopped leftover
cooked turkey and
add it just before
puréeing.

For a simple risotto,
stir into cooked
rice with a little
chicken stock.

1 tbsp	olive oil	15 mL
½ cup	diced peeled carrot	125 mL
½ cup	diced onion	125 mL
¼ cup	diced celery	50 mL
½ tsp	dried thyme	2 mL
6 oz	boneless skinless turkey breast, chopped	175 g
½ cup	low-sodium chicken stock	125 mL
¼ cup	fresh or frozen cranberries	50 mL

1. In a medium saucepan, heat oil over medium-high heat. Add carrot, onion, celery and thyme, stirring to combine. Cook, stirring, until vegetables are tender, about 5 minutes.

2. Add turkey and brown slightly. Stir in stock and cranberries, scraping any brown bits from bottom of pan; bring to a boil. Cover, reduce heat and simmer until cranberries are very tender and turkey is no longer pink inside, about 30 minutes. Let cool.

3. Transfer to blender and blend on high speed to desired consistency.

Nutritional Information (Per ½-cup/125 mL Serving)

Calories: 115 Kcal; Total Carbohydrates: 5 g; Fiber: 1 g; Fat: 6 g; Protein: 10 g; Iron: 1 mg

**MAKES ABOUT
2 CUPS (500 ML)**

TIP

For better flavor, substitute an equal amount of low-sodium beef stock for the water.

Beef

| 8 oz | lean ground sirloin beef | 250 g |
| 1 cup | water | 250 mL |

1. In a skillet, brown beef over medium-high heat, breaking up any large pieces, until no longer pink, about 7 minutes. Drain and let cool.

2. Transfer to blender, add water and purée on high speed.

Nutritional Information (Per ¼-cup/50 mL Serving)

Calories: 115 Kcal; Total Carbohydrates: 0 g; Fiber: 0 g; Fat: 8 g; Protein: 10 g; Iron: 1 mg

**MAKES ABOUT
2 CUPS (500 ML)**

FOR OLDER KIDS

Stir into cooked egg noodles for a simple weeknight meal.

Beefy Broccoli

6 oz	lean ground sirloin beef	175 g
2 cups	chopped broccoli florets and stems	500 mL
½ cup	low-sodium beef stock	125 mL

1. In a skillet, brown beef over medium-high heat, breaking up any large pieces, until no longer pink, about 7 minutes. Drain off fat and return beef to skillet.

2. Add broccoli and stock; cover, reduce heat and simmer until broccoli is very tender, about 15 minutes. Let cool.

3. Transfer to blender and blend on high speed to desired consistency.

Nutritional Information (Per ½-cup/125 mL Serving)

Calories: 85 Kcal; Total Carbohydrates: 3 g; Fiber: 1 g; Fat: 5 g; Protein: 8 g; Iron: 1 mg; Vitamin C: 41 mg

**MAKES ABOUT
2 CUPS (500 ML)**

*Carrots and orange
juice are the perfect
accompaniments
to beef.*

Beef with Carrots and Orange

6 oz	lean ground sirloin beef	175 g
1 cup	cubed peeled carrots (about 2)	250 mL
1 cup	unsweetened orange juice	250 mL

1. In a nonstick skillet, brown beef over medium-high heat, breaking up any large pieces, until no longer pink, about 7 minutes. Drain off fat and return beef to skillet.

2. Add carrots and orange juice; bring to a boil. Cover, reduce heat and simmer until carrots are very tender, about 20 minutes. Let cool.

3. Transfer to blender and blend on high speed to desired consistency.

Nutritional Information (Per ½-cup/125 mL Serving)

Calories: 141 Kcal; Total Carbohydrates: 10 g; Fiber: 1 g;
Fat: 7 g; Protein: 11 g; Iron: 1 mg; Vitamin C: 34 mg

**MAKES ABOUT
2 CUPS (500 ML)**

*Start this family
favorite from the
beginning!*

FOR OLDER KIDS

Spoon into a
hollowed-out whole
wheat dinner roll
and sprinkle with
shredded cheese. Bake
in preheated 350°F
(180°C) oven until
cheese is melted,
about 5 minutes.

Spoon ½ cup
(125 mL) chili onto
a split baked sweet
potato and sprinkle
with shredded
Cheddar cheese. Bake
in preheated 350°F
(180°C) oven until
cheese is melted and
potato is warmed
through, about
15 minutes. Top with
sour cream and sliced
green onions.

Chili for Beginners

6 oz	lean ground sirloin beef	175 g
1 cup	canned diced tomatoes, with juice	250 mL
½ cup	rinsed and drained canned red kidney beans	125 mL
¼ cup	diced green bell pepper	50 mL
¼ cup	frozen corn	50 mL

1. In a skillet, brown beef over medium-high heat, breaking up any large pieces, until no longer pink, about 7 minutes. Drain off fat and return beef to skillet.

2. Add tomatoes with juice, kidney beans, green pepper and corn. Cover, reduce heat and simmer for 15 minutes, until vegetables are very tender. Let cool.

3. Transfer to blender and blend on high speed to desired consistency.

Nutritional Information (Per ½-cup/125 mL Serving)

Calories: 117 Kcal; Total Carbohydrates: 10 g; Fiber: 3 g; Fat: 5 g; Protein: 8 g; Iron: 1 mg

**MAKES ABOUT
2 CUPS (500 ML)**

Shepherd's Pie

1	small Yukon gold potato, peeled and cubed	1
6 oz	lean ground sirloin beef	175 g
¼ cup	chopped onion	50 mL
¼ cup	chopped peeled carrot	50 mL
¼ cup	frozen peas	50 mL
¼ cup	frozen corn	50 mL

1. Place potato in a small saucepan of salted water and bring to a boil over medium-high heat; cook potato until tender, about 15 minutes. Drain.

2. Meanwhile, in a skillet, brown beef over medium-high heat, breaking up any large pieces, until no longer pink, about 7 minutes. Drain off fat and return to skillet. Add onion, carrot, peas and corn; cook, stirring occasionally, until onion and carrot are tender, about 10 minutes. Let cool.

3. Transfer to blender, add potato and blend on high speed to desired consistency.

Nutritional Information (Per ½-cup/125 mL Serving)

Calories: 117 Kcal; Total Carbohydrates: 9 g; Fiber: 2 g; Fat: 6 g; Protein: 7 g; Iron: 1 mg

MAKES ABOUT
2 CUPS (500 ML)

TIP

Add vegetable stock or more chicken stock to make a great soup for the whole family.

Ham and Split Peas

2 tsp	olive oil	10 mL
1	carrot, peeled and diced	1
1	celery stalk, diced	1
1/2	onion, diced	1/2
1/2 cup	diced cooked ham (about 4 oz/125 g)	125 mL
1 cup	low-sodium chicken stock	250 mL
1/2 cup	dried split yellow peas, rinsed	125 mL

1. In a medium saucepan, heat oil over medium-high heat. Add carrot, celery, onion and ham; cook, stirring occasionally, until carrots are tender, about 7 minutes.

2. Add stock and peas; cover, reduce heat and simmer until peas are tender, about 45 minutes. Let cool.

3. Transfer to blender and purée on high speed.

> **Nutritional Information (Per 1/2-cup/125 mL Serving)**
>
> Calories: 160 Kcal; Total Carbohydrates: 19 g; Fiber: 7 g; Fat: 4 g; Protein: 12 g; Iron: 2 mg

MAKES ABOUT
2 CUPS (500 ML)

Pork

8 oz	pork tenderloin, diced	250 g
1 cup	water	250 mL

1. In a medium saucepan, over medium heat, bring pork and water just to a boil. Cover, reduce heat and simmer until pork is no longer pink inside, about 15 minutes. Let cool.

2. Transfer to blender and purée on high speed.

> **Nutritional Information (Per 1/4-cup/50 mL Serving)**
>
> Calories: 68 Kcal; Total Carbohydrates: 0 g; Fiber: 0 g; Fat: 2 g; Protein: 12 g; Iron: 1 mg

**MAKES ABOUT
2 CUPS (500 ML)**

Babies like cabbage's mild flavor, and it stimulates the appetite and has antidiarrheal and antibiotic properties. It also stimulates flatulence, so feed it to your baby in moderation.

TIP

Golden Delicious apples are an ideal cooking apple because they retain their flavor when cooked.

Pork with Apples and Cabbage

1 tbsp	vegetable oil	15 mL
½ cup	diced onion	125 mL
8 oz	boneless pork loin chops, sliced	250 g
1	apple, peeled, cored and cubed	1
1 cup	shredded Savoy cabbage	250 mL
½ cup	sweetened apple juice or water (approx.)	125 mL

1. In a nonstick skillet, heat oil over medium-high heat. Add onion and cook, stirring, until tender but not browned, about 5 minutes. Add pork, turning to brown evenly. Add apple and cabbage; cook, stirring occasionally, for 5 minutes.

2. Pour apple juice into skillet; cover and cook, stirring occasionally, until cabbage and apple are very tender and pork is no longer pink inside, about 20 minutes. Let cool.

3. Transfer to blender and blend on high speed to desired consistency, adding more apple juice if necessary.

Nutritional Information (Per ½-cup/125 mL Serving)

Calories: 137 Kcal; Total Carbohydrates: 10 g; Fiber: 2 g; Fat: 6 g; Protein: 11 g; Iron: 1 mg

---

**MAKES ABOUT
2 CUPS (500 ML)**

*This purée is packed
full of fruit and fiber
to keep your little one
"moving"!*

TIP

If constipation is an
issue, increase the
prunes to ½ cup
(125 mL) and omit
the onions.

Pork with Prunes and Apples

¼ cup	pitted prunes	50 mL
½ cup	sweetened apple juice	125 mL
2 tsp	olive oil	10 mL
6 oz	boneless pork loin chop, sliced	175 g
¼ cup	sliced onion	50 mL
1	apple, peeled, cored and sliced	1

1. In a small bowl, pour apple juice over prunes; let sit for 15 minutes, until slightly softened.

2. Meanwhile, in a skillet, heat oil over medium-high heat. Add pork, turning to brown evenly. Transfer to a plate.

3. Add onion to skillet and cook, stirring, until tender and golden, about 5 minutes. Add apple and cook, stirring, for 5 minutes more. Stir in prunes with juice and browned pork; cover, reduce heat and simmer until apple and prunes are very tender and pork is no longer pink inside, about 10 minutes. Let cool.

4. Transfer to blender and blend on high speed to desired consistency.

Nutritional Information (Per ½-cup/125 mL Serving)

Calories: 120 Kcal; Total Carbohydrates: 16 g; Fiber: 2 g; Fat: 4 g; Protein: 6 g; Iron: 1 mg

---

Lamb has a distinct flavor that is softened by potatoes and peas.

Lamb with Mint, Peas and Potatoes

4 oz	lean ground lamb	125 g
1 cup	low-sodium beef stock	250 mL
½ cup	chopped peeled potato	125 mL
1 cup	frozen peas	250 mL
1 tbsp	chopped fresh mint	15 mL

1. In a medium saucepan, over medium-high heat, brown lamb until no pink remains, about 7 minutes. Drain and return to pan. Add stock and bring to a boil. Stir in potato and cook until tender, about 15 minutes. Add peas and mint; cook for 5 minutes more.

2. Transfer to blender and blend on high speed to desired consistency.

Variation

Substitute lean ground beef, chicken, turkey or pork for the lamb.

Nutritional Information (Per ½-cup/125 mL Serving)

Calories: 113 Kcal; Total Carbohydrates: 9 g; Fiber: 2 g; Fat: 2 g; Protein: 14 g; Iron: 2 mg

TIP

For a smoother, more "custard-like" consistency, use silken tofu. "Silken" refers to the texture, and it has a greater amount of liquid.

Tofu

1 cup	cubed firm tofu (about 4 oz/125 g)	250 mL

1. Place tofu in blender and purée on high speed.

Nutritional Information (Per ¼-cup/50 mL Serving)
Calories: 49 Kcal; Total Carbohydrates: 2 g; Fiber: 0 g; Fat: 3 g; Protein: 5 g; Iron: 1 mg

Adding tofu to fruit makes a simple complete meal without any fuss.

FOR OLDER KIDS

This recipe, or any recipe that combines silken tofu and puréed fruits, can help toddlers who avoid meat get some protein.

Apples, Plums and Tofu

2	plums, peeled and pitted	2
1 cup	unsweetened applesauce	250 mL
¼ cup	silken tofu (about 2 oz/60 g)	50 mL

1. In blender, on high speed, purée plums, applesauce and tofu.

Nutritional Information (Per ½-cup/125 mL Serving)
Calories: 55 Kcal; Total Carbohydrates: 11 g; Fiber: 1 g; Fat: 1 g; Protein: 2 g; Iron: 1 mg

**MAKES ABOUT
2 CUPS (500 ML)**

Apricots, Pears and Tofu

4	ripe apricots, stones removed	4
1	ripe pear, peeled and sliced	1
¼ cup	silken tofu (about 2 oz/60 g)	50 mL

1. In blender, on high speed, purée apricots, pear and tofu.

> **Nutritional Information (Per ½-cup/125 mL Serving)**
>
> Calories: 39 Kcal; Total Carbohydrates: 7 g; Fiber: 1 g; Fat: 1 g; Protein: 2 g; Iron: 1 mg

**MAKES ABOUT
2 CUPS (500 ML)**

This complete meal is nutritious and has a sweet, mellow flavor that babies love.

Butternut Squash, Corn and Tofu

1 cup	diced peeled butternut squash	250 mL
1 cup	low-sodium vegetable stock	250 mL
½ cup	frozen corn	125 mL
¼ cup	silken tofu (about 2 oz/60 g)	50 mL

1. In a medium saucepan, bring squash and stock to a boil over medium-high heat. Cover, reduce heat and simmer until squash is tender, about 20 minutes. Stir in corn and cook for 5 minutes more. Let cool.

2. Transfer to blender, add tofu and purée on high speed.

> **Nutritional Information (Per ½-cup/125 mL Serving)**
>
> Calories: 58 Kcal; Total Carbohydrates: 9 g; Fiber: 2 g; Fat: 1 g; Protein: 5 g; Iron: 2 mg

MAKES ABOUT 2 CUPS (500 ML)

Adding your own fruit purée to plain yogurt is a much healthier option than using store-bought varieties.

TIPS

The bacteria found in plain yogurt, called lactobacillus, works to maintain a balance in the intestinal tract. It is easy for little systems to digest. Avoid yogurts with preservatives, additives and coloring.

Avoid low-fat and no-fat dairy products for at least the first two years of your child's life. A child's brain needs fat for full development.

Lemon Raspberry Yogurt

½ cup	fresh or frozen raspberries	125 mL
1 ½ cup	vanilla-flavored yogurt	375 mL
	Grated zest and juice of 1 lemon	

1. In blender, on high speed, purée raspberries, yogurt, lemon zest and lemon juice.

2. *Make ahead:* Store in the refrigerator for up to 1 week.

Variation

Use an equal amount of any fruit you have on hand for a different flavor every day.

Nutritional Information (Per ¼-cup/50 mL Serving)

Calories: 34 Kcal; Total Carbohydrates: 4 g; Fiber: 1 g; Fat: 2 g; Protein: 2 g; Iron: 0 mg

**MAKES ABOUT
2 CUPS (500 ML)**

FOR OLDER KIDS

Serve over pound cake.

Over-the-Top Applesauce

4 cups	sliced peeled Golden Delicious apples (about 5)	1 L
½ cup	unsweetened apple juice	125 mL
¼ cup	ricotta or mascarpone cheese	50 mL
1 tsp	ground cinnamon	5 mL
½ tsp	grated lemon zest	2 mL
¼ tsp	ground ginger	1 mL
¼ tsp	ground nutmeg	1 mL

1. In a medium saucepan, combine apples with apple juice. Cover and simmer until apples break down and are very tender.

2. Transfer to blender and add ricotta, cinnamon, lemon zest, ginger and nutmeg; purée on high speed.

3. *Make ahead:* Store in the refrigerator for up to 1 week.

Nutritional Information (Per ¼-cup/50 mL Serving)

Calories: 46 Kcal; Total Carbohydrates: 8 g; Fiber: 1 g; Fat: 1 g; Protein: 1 g; Iron: 0 mg

*Cherries make
everyday bananas out
of this world!*

TIP

Substitute jarred sour
cherries when you
cannot find fresh
or frozen.

FOR OLDER KIDS

This makes a great
smoothie for older
children — and
adults too!

Banana Cherry Blast

1	very ripe banana	1
½ cup	pitted sour cherries	125 mL
¼ cup	cherry juice (drained from cherries)	50 mL
½ cup	plain yogurt	125 mL

1. In blender, on high speed, purée banana, cherries, cherry juice and yogurt.

2. *Make ahead:* Store in the refrigerator for up to 3 days. Do not freeze.

Nutritional Information (Per ½-cup/125 mL Serving)

Calories: 149 Kcal; Total Carbohydrates: 31 g; Fiber: 2 g;
Fat: 2 g; Protein: 3 g; Iron: 0 mg

*Mild, creamy polenta
blends beautifully with
apricots and yogurt.*

Polenta with Apricots

½ cup	dried apricots, chopped	125 mL
1½ cups	low-sodium chicken stock	375 mL
½ cup	cornmeal	125 mL
¼ cup	plain yogurt	50 mL

1. In a medium saucepan, bring apricots and chicken stock to a boil. Gradually stir in cornmeal until well combined. Reduce heat and simmer, stirring frequently, until mixture is creamy. Let cool slightly.

2. Transfer to blender, add yogurt and purée on high speed.

**MAKES ABOUT
2 CUPS (500 ML)**

FOR OLDER KIDS

This makes a great sandwich spread, with extra slices of banana in between slices of whole wheat bread.

Avocado, Banana and Yogurt

1	banana	1
1	avocado, peeled and pitted	1
½ cup	plain yogurt	125 mL

1. In blender, on high speed, purée banana, avocado and yogurt.
2. *Make ahead:* Store in the refrigerator for up to 3 days. Do not freeze.

Nutritional Information (Per ¼-cup/50 mL Serving)

Calories: 65 Kcal; Total Carbohydrates: 9 g; Fiber: 1 g; Fat: 3 g; Protein: 1 g; Iron: 0 mg

**MAKES ABOUT
2 CUPS (500 ML)**

Fruity Cottage Cheese

½ cup	canned mandarin orange segments, drained and rinsed	125 mL
½ cup	sliced strawberries	125 mL
½ cup	sliced peach	125 mL
½ cup	2% cottage cheese	125 mL
¼ cup	unsweetened peach nectar	50 mL

1. In blender, on high speed, purée oranges, strawberries, peach, cottage cheese and peach nectar.
2. *Make ahead:* Store in the refrigerator for up to 3 days. Do not freeze.

Nutritional Information (Per ¼-cup/50 mL Serving)

Calories: 30 Kcal; Total Carbohydrates: 5 g; Fiber: 1 g; Fat: 0 g; Protein: 2 g; Iron: 0 mg

**MAKES ABOUT
2 CUPS (500 ML)**

FOR OLDER KIDS

Serve as a dip with celery sticks and pieces of apple and pear.

Mango, Banana and Cottage Cheese

1	banana	1
1	mango, peeled, pitted and cubed	1
½ cup	small-curd cottage cheese	125 mL

1. In blender, on high speed, purée banana, mango and cottage cheese.

2. *Make ahead:* Store in the refrigerator for up to 3 days. Do not freeze.

> **Nutritional Information (Per ¼-cup/50 mL Serving)**
>
> Calories: 43 Kcal; Total Carbohydrates: 8 g; Fiber: 1 g; Fat: 0 g; Protein: 2 g; Iron: 0 mg

**MAKES ABOUT
2 CUPS (500 ML)**

Adding cottage cheese to vegetables makes for a protein-rich meal.

Sweet Potato and Cottage Cheese

2 cups	cubed peeled sweet potatoes (about 2 small)	500 mL
½ cup	unsweetened apple juice	125 mL
½ cup	small-curd cottage cheese	125 mL

1. Arrange sweet potatoes in a steamer basket fitted over a medium saucepan of boiling water. Cover and steam until potatoes are very tender, about 20 minutes. Let cool.

2. Transfer to blender and add apple juice and cottage cheese; purée on high speed.

> **Nutritional Information (Per ¼-cup/50 mL Serving)**
>
> Calories: 46 Kcal; Total Carbohydrates: 8 g; Fiber: 1 g; Fat: 0 g; Protein: 2 g; Iron: 0 mg

MAKES ABOUT 2 CUPS (500 ML)

Creamy ricotta balances the acidity of spinach and tomatoes.

TIPS

Fresh spinach is very sandy and must be washed thoroughly in a large basin of water. Change the water if necessary. Trim woody stems for even cooking.

Steaming spinach tends to bring out its bitterness. Instead, cook it in a covered saucepan, over high heat, in the liquid that remains on the leaves after washing.

FOR OLDER KIDS

Stir into cooked pasta.

Spinach and Tomatoes with Ricotta

1 tbsp	olive oil	15 mL
1	clove garlic, minced	1
1/2 cup	canned diced tomatoes, with juice	125 mL
2 cups	trimmed spinach	500 mL
1/4 cup	ricotta cheese	50 mL
2 tsp	freshly squeezed lemon juice	10 mL

1. In a skillet, heat oil over medium heat. Add garlic and tomatoes with juice; cook until garlic is fragrant but not browned, about 2 minutes. Stir in spinach and cook until completely wilted, about 3 minutes. Let cool.

2. Transfer to blender and add ricotta and lemon juice; purée on high speed.

Nutritional Information (Per 1/4-cup/50 mL Serving)

Calories: 35 Kcal; Total Carbohydrates: 3 g; Fiber: 0 g; Fat: 3 g; Protein: 1 g; Iron: 0 mg

---

**MAKES ABOUT
2 CUPS (500 ML)**

*Cauliflower is the
most easily digestible
member of the
cabbage family and
is an excellent
source of vitamin C
and potassium.*

Tomato, Cauliflower and Cheese

2 tsp	olive oil	10 mL
1/4 cup	chopped onion	50 mL
1 cup	cauliflower florets	250 mL
1/2 cup	canned diced tomatoes, with juice	125 mL
1/4 cup	shredded Cheddar cheese	50 mL

1. In a skillet, heat oil over medium-high heat. Add onion and cook, stirring occasionally, until tender, but not browned, about 5 minutes. Add cauliflower and tomatoes with juice. Cover, reduce heat and simmer until cauliflower is tender, about 10 minutes. Let cool.

2. Transfer to blender, add cheese and purée on high speed.

Nutritional Information (Per 1/4-cup/50 mL Serving)

Calories: 32 Kcal; Total Carbohydrates: 2 g; Fiber: 1 g;
Fat: 2 g; Protein: 1 g; Iron: 0 mg

**MAKES ABOUT
2 CUPS (500 ML)**

*Cauliflower mellows
out the flavor of
broccoli without
compromising
nutrients or taste.*

TIP

To increase the fiber
content of vegetable
dishes, sprinkle with
1 tbsp (15 mL) wheat
germ before puréeing.
To maintain its
freshness, store wheat
germ in an airtight
container in the
refrigerator for up
to 6 months or in
the freezer for up
to 1 year.

Broccoli and Cauliflower Gratin

1 cup	broccoli florets	250 mL
1 cup	cauliflower florets	250 mL
1 cup	low-sodium vegetable stock	250 mL
½ cup	shredded Cheddar cheese	125 mL

1. In a medium saucepan, combine broccoli, cauliflower and vegetable stock; bring to a boil. Cover, reduce heat and simmer until vegetables are very tender, about 15 minutes. Let cool.

2. Transfer to blender, add cheese and purée on high speed.

Nutritional Information (Per ¼-cup/50 mL Serving)

Calories: 40 Kcal; Total Carbohydrates: 1 g; Fiber: 1 g;
Fat: 2 g; Protein: 4 g; Iron: 0 mg

**MAKES ABOUT
2 CUPS (500 ML)**

Fisherman's Pie

1	small Yukon gold potato, peeled and cubed	1
¼ cup	chopped onion	50 mL
4 oz	trout fillet (skin removed)	125 g
½ cup	frozen corn	125 mL
½ cup	broccoli florets	125 mL
¼ cup	shredded Cheddar cheese	50 mL

1. Place potato in a small saucepan of salted water. Bring to a boil over medium-high heat and cook until potato is tender, about 15 minutes. Drain.

2. Meanwhile, in a skillet, heat oil over medium-high heat. Add onion and cook until tender, about 5 minutes. Add trout, browning on both sides. Stir in corn and broccoli; cover and cook until fish flakes easily when pierced with a fork and broccoli is tender, about 5 minutes. Let cool.

3. Transfer to blender and add potatoes and cheese; blend on high speed to desired consistency.

Nutritional Information (Per ½-cup/125 mL Serving)

Calories: 63 Kcal; Total Carbohydrates: 12 g; Fiber: 1 g; Fat: 0 g; Protein: 4 g; Iron: 1 mg

---

**MAKES ABOUT
2 CUPS (500 ML)**

*This quick skillet
supper is good for
every age!*

Cheesy Beef Casserole

6 oz	lean ground sirloin beef	175 g
¼ cup	chopped onion	50 mL
½ cup	chopped peeled carrot	125 mL
1 cup	canned diced tomatoes, with juice	250 mL
½ cup	shredded Cheddar cheese	125 mL
	Water (optional)	

1. In a skillet, brown beef over medium-high heat, breaking up any large pieces, until no longer pink, about 5 minutes. Drain off fat and return beef to skillet. Add onion, carrot and tomatoes with juice. Cover and cook, stirring occasionally, until onion and carrot are tender, about 10 minutes. Let cool.

2. Transfer to blender, add cheese and blend on high speed to desired consistency, adding water if necessary.

Nutritional Information (Per ½-cup/125 mL Serving)

Calories: 200 Kcal; Total Carbohydrates: 7 g; Fiber: 1 g; Fat: 13 g; Protein: 15 g; Iron: 2 mg

---

**MAKES ABOUT
2 CUPS (500 ML)**

*Kids can't get enough
pasta, so get in the
habit of making simple
pasta dishes and avoid
packaged varieties.*

Cheesy Broccoli and Ham Pasta

½ cup	pastini	125 mL
1 cup	broccoli florets	250 mL
½ cup	diced cooked ham (about 4 oz/125 g)	125 mL
½ cup	herb-flavored cream cheese	125 mL

1. Add pastini and broccoli to a saucepan of boiling water; cook until tender, about 10 minutes. Drain, reserving ¼ cup (50 mL) of the cooking liquid. Stir in ham, cream cheese and reserved cooking liquid until well combined.

2. Transfer to blender and blend on high speed to desired consistency.

Nutritional Information (Per ½-cup/125 mL Serving)

Calories: 206 Kcal; Total Carbohydrates: 12 g; Fiber: 1 g; Fat: 13 g; Protein: 9 g; Iron: 1 mg; Vitamin C: 24 mg

**MAKES ABOUT
2 CUPS (500 ML)**

*Smoothies are an
excellent way to pack
extra vitamins and
nutrients into your
child's day.*

TIP

Use whole oranges
in place of juice
whenever possible.
Make sure to remove
peel, pith and seeds,
which are bitter.

Orange Banana Smoothie

1	banana	1
1 cup	sliced peeled orange (about 1)	250 mL

1. In blender, on high speed, purée banana and orange.

Nutritional Information (Per ¼-cup/50 mL Serving)

Calories: 101 Kcal; Total Carbohydrates: 26 g; Fiber: 3 g;
Fat: 0 g; Protein: 1 g; Iron: 0 mg

**MAKES ABOUT
1 CUP (250 ML)**

*This recipe can be
mixed with formula
or with any fruit or
vegetable purée to
increase fiber intake.
Try it in Blueberry
Apricot Crumble or
Blue Nectarine Yogurt
(see recipes, page 361).*

TIP

This recipe is suitable
for babies 9 months
and older if the
almonds are omitted.

Mixed Grains

● *Preheat oven to 350°F (180°C)*
● *Rimmed baking sheet*

1 cup	old-fashioned rolled oats	250 mL
¼ cup	bran cereal	50 mL
¼ cup	unblanched almonds (optional)	50 mL
2 tbsp	wheat germ	25 mL

1. Spread oats, bran cereal, almonds (if using) and wheat
germ on baking sheet. Bake in preheated oven until
fragrant and lightly toasted, about 7 minutes. Let cool.

2. Transfer toasted grains to blender and purée on
high speed.

3. *Make ahead:* Store in a cool place for up to 1 month.

Nutritional Information (Per ¼-cup/50 mL Serving)

Calories: 158 Kcal; Total Carbohydrates: 22 g; Fiber: 6 g;
Fat: 6 g; Protein: 6 g; Iron: 2 mg

Blueberry Apricot Crumble

MAKES ABOUT 2 CUPS (500 ML)

These two fruits are nutritional dynamos and provide a wonderful meal when combined with energy-boosting grains.

TIP

When apricots are not in season, substitute dried apricots. Soak them in hot water to soften.

1 1/2 cups	sliced pitted apricots (4 to 5)	375 mL
1/2 cup	frozen wild blueberries, thawed	125 mL
1/4 cup	orange juice	50 mL
1/2 cup	Mixed Grains (see recipe, page 360)	125 mL

1. In blender, on high speed, purée apricots, blueberries and orange juice.
2. Sprinkle with Mixed Grains. For softer grains, let sit for 5 minutes before serving.

Nutritional Information (Per 1/4-cup/50 mL Serving)

Calories: 59 Kcal; Total Carbohydrates: 9 g; Fiber: 2 g; Fat: 2 g; Protein: 2 g; Iron: 0 mg

Blue Nectarine Yogurt

MAKES ABOUT 2 CUPS (500 ML)

Cereals based on oats provide long-lasting energy throughout the day. Mix them with your child's favorite fruit, yogurt or cottage cheese to get them through action-packed days.

TIP

Add milk to each serving as desired for a thinner consistency.

1 cup	sliced nectarines (about 2)	250 mL
1/4 cup	fresh or thawed frozen blueberries	50 mL
1 cup	plain yogurt	250 mL
1 cup	Mixed Grains (see recipe, page 360)	250 mL

1. In blender, on high speed, purée nectarines and blueberries.
2. Transfer to a medium bowl and stir in yogurt.
3. For each serving, mix 1/4 cup (50 mL) yogurt mixture with 2 tbsp (25 mL) Mixed Grains. Let sit for 5 minutes before serving.

Nutritional Information (Per 1/4-cup/50 mL Serving)

Calories: 136 Kcal; Total Carbohydrates: 18 g; Fiber: 4 g; Fat: 5 g; Protein: 5 g; Iron: 0 mg

**MAKES ABOUT
2 CUPS (500 ML)**

*Raspberries and
blueberries are packed
with nutrients, but are
too strong to offer to
your baby on their
own. Adding a few into
pears is an economical,
tasty solution.*

TIP

This recipe is suitable
for babies six months
and older if the honey
is omitted.

FOR OLDER KIDS

Turn ordinary
porridge into
something special
by mixing in some
of this purée, along
with a sprinkle of
toasted almonds.

Very Berry Pears

3 cups	diced peeled pears (about 4)	750 mL
½ cup	water (approx.)	125 mL
¼ cup	raspberries	50 mL
¼ cup	blueberries	50 mL
1 tbsp	liquid honey (optional)	15 mL

1. In a medium saucepan, over medium-low heat, combine pears, water, raspberries, blueberries and honey (if using). Cover and simmer, stirring occasionally, until pears are very tender, about 30 minutes. Let cool.

2. Transfer to blender and purée on high speed, adding more water if necessary.

Nutritional Information (Per ¼-cup/50 mL Serving)

Calories: 44 Kcal; Total Carbohydrates: 11 g; Fiber: 2 g; Fat: 0 g; Protein: 0 g; Iron: 0 mg

**MAKES ABOUT
2 CUPS (500 ML)**

*Get in the habit of
sprinkling wheat germ
over all your veggies
to sneak in some
extra fiber.*

TIP

Toasting nuts, seeds
and grains brings out
their flavor. Toast
them on a rimmed
baking sheet in a
350°F (180°C) oven
until fragrant and
lightly golden, about
5 minutes. Let cool
before using.

Broccoli and Cauliflower Melt

1 cup	broccoli florets and peeled stems	250 mL
1 cup	cauliflower florets	250 mL
1 cup	homogenized (whole) milk	250 mL
2 tbsp	toasted old-fashioned rolled oats	25 mL
1 tbsp	wheat germ	15 mL
½ cup	shredded Cheddar cheese	125 mL

1. In a medium saucepan, over medium-high heat, combine broccoli, cauliflower, milk, oats and wheat germ; bring to a boil. Cover, reduce heat and simmer until vegetables are very tender, about 20 minutes. Stir in cheese. Let cool.

2. Transfer to blender and purée on high speed.

Nutritional Information (Per ¼-cup/50 mL Serving)

Calories: 61 Kcal; Total Carbohydrates: 4 g; Fiber: 1 g; Fat: 4 g; Protein: 4 g; Iron: 0 mg

**MAKES ABOUT
2 CUPS (500 ML)**

Broccoli Bake

- *Preheat oven to 350°F (180°C)*
- *8-inch (2 L) square baking dish, greased*

2 cups	frozen broccoli florets and stems	500 mL
½ cup	shredded Cheddar cheese	125 mL
¼ cup	Mixed Grains (see recipe, page 360)	50 mL

1. Place broccoli in a colander; run under hot water for 30 seconds and drain well.

2. Arrange broccoli in baking dish. Sprinkle with cheese and Mixed Grains; cover with foil. Bake in preheated oven until broccoli is tender and cheese is melted, about 20 minutes. Remove foil and bake for 5 minutes more, until grains are golden.

3. Transfer to blender and blend on high speed to desired consistency.

Nutritional Information (Per ¼-cup/50 mL Serving)

Calories: 52 Kcal; Total Carbohydrates: 4 g; Fiber: 2 g;
Fat: 3 g; Protein: 3 g; Iron: 0 mg

**MAKES 2 CUPS
(500 ML)**

*Sometimes we have to
be a bit sneaky when
our toddlers are going
through a "non-veggie"
stage . . . what they
don't know can be good
for them!*

TIP

Use this sauce in any
recipe that calls for
prepared pasta sauce.

Veggie Red Sauce

1 tbsp	olive oil	15 mL
1	clove garlic, minced	1
1 cup	chopped peeled carrots (about 2)	250 mL
½ cup	chopped peeled broccoli stems	125 mL
¼ cup	chopped onion	50 mL
1 cup	canned diced tomatoes, with juice	250 mL

1. In a skillet, heat oil over medium-high heat. Add garlic, carrots, broccoli stems and onion and stir to combine. Cook, stirring, until carrots are tender, about 7 minutes. Add tomatoes with juice, reduce heat and simmer until vegetables are very tender, about 15 minutes. Let cool.

2. Transfer to blender and purée on high speed.

Nutritional Information (Per ¼-cup/50 mL Serving)

Calories: 33 Kcal; Total Carbohydrates: 4 g; Fiber: 1 g;
Fat: 2 g; Protein: 1 g; Iron: 0 mg

**MAKES ABOUT
2 CUPS (500 ML)**

Try this sauce over pastini or stirred into any meat purée to boost nutritional value and flavor.

Veggie Cream Sauce

1 tbsp	olive oil	15 mL
1 cup	peeled and diced carrots (about 2)	250 mL
½ cup	diced peeled broccoli stem	125 mL
¼ cup	diced onion	50 mL
1	clove garlic, minced	1
2 tbsp	cubed softened cream cheese	25 mL
1 cup	low-sodium chicken stock	250 mL

1. In a skillet, heat oil over medium-high heat. Stir in carrots, broccoli, onion and garlic; cook, stirring often, until carrots are tender, about 5 minutes. Whisk in cream cheese and stock; bring just to a boil. Reduce heat and simmer, uncovered, until vegetables are very tender, about 10 minutes. Let cool.

2. Transfer to blender and purée on high speed.

Nutritional Information (Per ¼-cup/50 mL Serving)

Calories: 33 Kcal; Total Carbohydrates: 4 g; Fiber: 1 g; Fat: 2 g; Protein: 1 g; Iron: 0 mg

---

Library and Archives Canada Cataloguing in Publication

Chase, Andrew
    The blender bible / Andrew Chase & Nicole Young.

Includes index.
ISBN 0-7788-0109-8

1. Blenders (Cookery) I. Young, Nicole II. Title.

TX840.B5C43 2005   641.5'893   C2004-906510-6

General Index

G

Garam Masala, 147
garlic
  Aioli, 59
  Almond and Garlic
    Gazpacho, 123
  Anchovy Pistou, 61
  Anchovy Spread, 29
  Asparagus Soup with
    Frizzled Prosciutto, 129
  Bagna Cauda, 29
  Beef in New Mexico Red
    Chili Sauce, 154
  Black Bean Soup, 87
  Caesar Salad Dressing, 46
  Chicken and Cashew
    Coconut Curry, 150
  Chicken Liver Pâté, 31
  Chicken Mole, 144
  Chicken Tandoori, 146
  Chicken Tikka, 148
  Chili Vinegar Sauce, 70
  Classic Tomato Ketchup, 48
  Cold Spinach and Parsley
    Soup, 116
  Collard Green and Sausage
    Soup, 130
  Cream of Spinach Soup, 115
  Curried Pumpkin Dip, 19
  Fennel Tomato Soup, 120
  Four-Lily Vichyssoise, 114
  Fresh Tomato Sauce, 63
  Garlic Dressing, 37
  Garlic Soup, 98
  Goan Fish Curry, 159
  Kale and Bread Soup, 99
  Lemon Grass Chicken, 149
  Lightened-Up Garlic
    Dressing, 38
  Mushroom Dip, 22
  Olive and Garlic Dip, 15
  Onion and Garlic Dip, 15
  Oven-Baked Ribs with Latin
    Spice Rub, 157
  Pesto, 60
  Potato-Parsley Soup, 108
  Red Pepper Rouille, 77
  Roasted Carrot and Parsnip
    Dip, 21
  Roasted Garlic and Rosemary
    Dressing, 39
  Roasted Garlic Dip, 20
  Saffron Rouille, 77
  Scotch Bonnet Hot Sauce, 71
  Shrimp Balchao, 164
  Spanish Garlic Soup, 98
  Spanish Tomato Gazpacho,
    122

Thai Cooked Chili Sauce, 73
Thai Green Curry Paste, 80
Thai Massaman Curry Paste,
  82
Thai Red Curry Paste, 81
Tomatillos Ketchup, 49
Vietnamese Mekong Shrimp,
  163
Gazpacho Smoothie, 210
gin
  Après les Huîtres, 255
  Blue Lagoon, 265
  Gin Fizz, 262
  Green Goddess, 254
  La Vie en Rose, 254
  Pink Gin Whizz, 255
  Pink Greyhound, 255
  Raspberry Martini, 256
  Sapphire Fizz, 264
  Watermelon and Basil
    Martini, 257
  Watermelon Martini, 256
  White Cargo, 273
  Winter Greyhound, 254
Gingery Parsnip Soup, 108
Goan Fish Curry, 159
Gout Potion, 279
Grape Blueberry Fizz, 223
grapefruit
  Citrus and Rum Mousse, 190
  Ruby Red Smoothie, 214
grapefruit juice
  Pink Greyhound, 255
  Pink Whippet, 253
  Winter Greyhound, 254
  Winter Whippet, 252
Green Goddess, 254
Green Smoothie, 211
Green Spring Soup, 102
Green Tea "Milkshake," 219
greens. See also spinach; Swiss
  chard
  Blender Beet Borscht, 88
  Collard Green and Sausage
    Soup, 130
Guinness Punch, 238
Gypsy Rose, 250

H

Hair of the Clam, 280
Hamlet's Blood, 261
Harissa, 72
Hazelnut Torte, 193
Herbed Yogurt Cheese, 16
Hollandaise Sauce, 58
Homemade Rice Milk, 230
Horseradish Mustard,
  Seed-Style, 53

Hot Honey Mustard, 52
Hot Honeydew Freezie, 251
Hot Pink Ginger, 252
Hot Watermelon Freezie, 252
Hummus, Quick, 24

I

Iced Coffee Frappé, 233
Indonesian Spicy Tomato
  Sauce, 66
Irish Cream Coffee, 275
Italian Spinach, 167
Italian-Style Ricotta
  Cheesecake, 194

J

Jack Splat, 277
Jamaican Dirty Banana, 240
Jelly, Rhubarb and Strawberry,
  192
Jerk Marinade, 153
Jerusalem Artichoke Soup, 85

K

Kale and Bread Soup, 99
ketchups, 48–51
Kipper Pâté, 27
kirsch. See brandy, flavored

L

La Vie en Rose, 254
lamb. See beef and lamb
lassi drinks, 225–27
Latin Spice Rub, 157
leeks
  Cheddar and Beer Soup, 127
  Cheddar Cheese Soup, 125
  Cream of Mushroom Soup,
    105
  Leek and Swiss Chard Soup,
    101
  Smoked Haddock Soup, 132
  Vichyssoise, 114
lemon
  Apple Butter, 204
  Blueberry Lemonade, 224
  Cold Blueberry Soup, 180
  Italian-Style Ricotta
    Cheesecake, 194
  Lemon Sauce, 205
  Lemony Eggplant Dip, 17
  No-Bake Lemon Cheesecake,
    195
  Papaya Lemon Grass Sorbet,
    183

White Cargo, 273
White Chocolate Cheesecake, 196
White Chocolate Coconut Sauce, 208
White Flour Blinis, 11
White Russian Shake, 274
White Turnip Soup, 117
White Wine–Tarragon Mustard, 52
wine
   Blender Bellini, 268
   Blueberry Sparkler, 270
   Cold Blueberry Soup, 180
   Cuc'a Sake Martini, 260
   Egg Flip, 229
   Mango Sparkler, 271
   Peach Sparkler, 270
   Persimmon Sparkler, 271
   Pineapple Sparkler, 271

Raspberry Peach Sparkler, 270
Rhubarb and Strawberry Jelly, 192
White Wine–Tarragon Mustard, 52
Winter Celery Root Soup, 93
Winter Greyhound, 254
Winter Whippet, 252

Y

Yellow Tomato Sauce, 166
yogurt. *See also* yogurt, vanilla-flavored
   Avocado Dressing, 35
   Chicken Tandoori, 146
   Cold Cucumber Soup, 95
   Cucumber Dressing, 35
   Cucumber Yogurt Sauce, 69

Cucumber Yogurt Smoothie, 211
Curried Pumpkin Dip, 19
Herbed Yogurt Cheese, 16
Mango Ginger Smoothie, 215
Mango Lassi, 227
Ruby Red Smoothie, 214
Salty Lassi, 226
Sweet Lassi, 225
Tomato Lassi, 226
yogurt, vanilla-flavored
   Apple Apricot Smoothie, 213
   Blueberry Smoothie, 213
   Grape Blueberry Fizz, 223
   Lime Frost, 223
   Neapolitan Smoothie, 216
   Pink Berry Smoothie, 213
   Strawberry Freeze, 189
Yorkshire Puddings, 171

Baby Food Index

Also Available
from Robert Rose

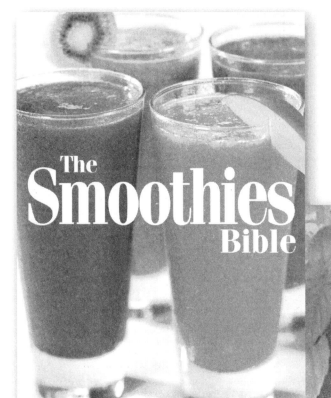

The
Smoothies
Bible

Pat Crocker

THE **Juicing** BIBLE

PAT CROCKER
& SUSAN EAGLES

Robert
ROSE